Dr Ante Bilić
liječnik - stomatolog

09. 04. 1981
Ante Bilić

Introduction to Oral Medicine

Introduction to Oral Medicine

DERRICK M. CHISHOLM, BDS, PhD, FDS

*Professor of Dental Surgery, University of Dundee, Dundee;
Formerly Senior Lecturer in Oral Medicine and Pathology,
University of Glasgow, Glasgow*

MARTIN M. FERGUSON, BSc, MB, ChB, BDS, FDS

*Lecturer in Oral Medicine and Pathology,
Glasgow Dental Hospital and School,
University of Glasgow, Glasgow*

J. HAROLD JONES, MD, MSc, FRCPath, FFD

*Professor of Oral Medicine, The Turner Dental School,
University of Manchester, Manchester*

DAVID K. MASON, BDS, MD, FDS, FRCS, FRCPath

*Professor of Oral Medicine and Pathology,
Glasgow Dental Hospital and School,
University of Glasgow, Glasgow*

1978

W. B. Saunders Company Ltd   London · Philadelphia · Toronto

W. B. Saunders Company Ltd: 1 St Anne's Road
                          Eastbourne, East Sussex BN21 3UN

                          West Washington Square
                          Philadelphia, PA 19105

                          1 Goldthorne Avenue
                          Toronto, Ontario M8Z 5T9

Library of Congress Cataloging in Publication Data

Main entry under title:

Introduction to oral medicine.

   Includes bibliographies.
   1. Mouth—Diseases.   2. Oral manifestations of general diseases.
3. Teeth—Diseases.   I. Chisholm, Derrick M.
   [DNLM: 1. Mouth diseases—diagnosis.   2. Mouth diseases—Therapy.
WU140 I61]
RC815.I58   617'.522   77-91849

ISBN 0-7216-2593-2

Printed at The Lavenham Press Ltd, Lavenham, Suffolk, England.

Print No: 9 8 7 6 5 4 3 2 1

PREFACE

By tradition and of necessity, the clinical dental undergraduate curriculum has been mainly concerned with surgical and other practical techniques aimed at the treatment of disease and the restoration of function.

In recent years there have been considerable developments in our knowledge of oral disease. It is clear that patients with these conditions may need several detailed investigations and that the clinicians concerned require special knowledge of the diseases, their differential diagnosis and treatment. This book seeks to present the physician's approach to the diagnosis, management and treatment of oral disease. It is written primarily for undergraduate dental students, general dental practitioners and medical practitioners, and links many aspects of medicine and dentistry.

Chapters on the structure, development and function of the normal oral tissues are included principally for the medical and non-dental reader. They may also serve as a convenient source of revision for the student of dentistry.

Although the authors recognize the need for a sound knowledge of oral pathology in the practice of oral medicine, they have deliberately excluded detailed descriptions and illustrations of histopathology: information of this nature is readily available in established text books, some of which are alluded to in the further reading lists provided at the end of the chapters.

ACKNOWLEDGEMENTS

We have much pleasure in acknowledging the help we have received from many of our colleagues, in particular Professor M. R. Bond, Dr W. N. Mason, Mr K. W. Stephen, Mr D. Stenhouse, Mr T. W. Macfarlane and Dr D. A. M. Geddes. We would also like to thank colleagues with whom we have worked closely over the years: Dr J. H. Dagg, Dr A. Lyell, Professor W. W. Buchanan and Dr W. D. Alexander.

To the late Professor J. A. Milne and Dr I. Pinkerton we gratefully acknowledge a number of illustrations of dermatological and childhood infective disease. For additional illustrations we thank Professor H. Dean Millard, Dr D. G. MacDonald, Mr H. Critchlow and Professor D. A. McGowan.

Our thanks are due to Churchill Livingstone for permission to publish Table 19.1 which is modified from Schour and Massler (1940) and Kraus (1959), and is taken from Scott and Symons, *Introduction to Dental Anatomy*.

To Mr John Davis and his Staff in the Department of Medical Illustration, Glasgow Dental Hospital and School, we gratefully acknowledge the preparation of photographs, line drawings and diagrams. It gives us much pleasure to thank Mrs I. McGuire, Miss J. McLeod and Miss H. Sugden who typed the manuscript and gave unfailing help and assistance.

Finally, we wish to thank Mr David Inglis and the Staff of W. B. Saunders Company Ltd for their help, encouragement and assistance.

D. M. CHISHOLM
M. M. FERGUSON
J. H. JONES
D. K. MASON

v

CONTENTS

Appendices   275

part 1

GENERAL CONSIDERATIONS

chapter 1

Introduction and General Considerations

The Physician's Approach
Oral and Systemic Disease
The Roles of Dentist, Doctor and Hospital Specialist
Referral of Patients
The Oral Medicine Clinic

THE PHYSICIAN'S APPROACH

Dentistry in Europe and in North America became a learned profession in the middle of the nineteenth century, and from the beginning, in its creation and development, was associated with surgery. At the present time, the dental undergraduate curriculum, in contrast to its medical counterpart, is largely devoted to patient care with clinical treatment which is mainly surgical in character. In consequence, dentists tend to have a 'surgical approach' to their patients' problems.

Historically, the surgeon differed from the physician in training and function. The surgeon was intensely practical in approach, using physical means, chiefly 'cutting', to eradicate diseased or damaged tissues. The physician's art was based on the philosophies and knowledge, or, perhaps more correctly, the tradition, maintained in the great universities and other centres of learning, and changed little over many centuries. In the last 200 years the surgeon's practical approach has been increasingly based on careful research and training and the physician's art has developed into a science. There remains this difference, however: the surgeon tends to employ physical techniques, and the physician drugs, to treat disease. It follows that the surgeon often quickly finishes with a case, having removed the diseased part, but the physician's approach may involve more prolonged treatment and observation. Nowadays, both rely on scientific investigation and basic research but differences in training programmes and in the facilities required for the practice of surgery and medicine persist.

Dentistry remains an intensely practical discipline and much time is devoted to the acquisition of manual skills in training. The qualified dentist devotes the main part of his time to surgical procedures in the mouth. Notable exceptions are in orthodontics

3

and in prosthodontics where non-surgical skills, although they still involve practical procedures, are employed. Dentists have become increasingly aware of the broad concept of oral health. It was found that systemic factors frequently influence oral tissues, and this has encouraged an investigative approach which parallels that of the physician. They have appreciated that many of the diseases which are considered 'medical' rather than 'surgical' have important consequences in the mouth. These trends have involved the emergence of oral physicians to practise alongside oral surgeons in some of the major teaching hospitals, although elsewhere both approaches are practised in one department. In the dental context, the oral physician is concerned with all aspects of general medicine, in the way in which these may relate to the mouth. More detailed consideration of the requirements for the practice of oral medicine are given later in this chapter (see 'The Oral Medicine Clinic') and the methods of diagnosis receive attention in Chapter 2.

It may be helpful at this stage to consider some simple examples which illustrate the difference between surgeon and physician in dentistry. A fractured jaw with displacement clearly requires a surgical approach — in most cases early reduction and immobilization are necessary. The same may be said of an apical abscess which requires extraction of the tooth, although the surgeon will pay due regard to the patient's general health and the infection which is likely to be present. However, in both these instances practical 'surgical' intervention is required.

In contrast, the complaint of persistent dryness of the mouth, which usually results from degenerative disease of salivary glands, requires a physician's approach with full investigation of the patient and special tests involving salivary and lacrimal gland function. The programme of treatment and management does not necessitate surgical intervention, but long-term and prolonged supervision is essential. For oral ulceration, prompt biopsy or excision may be needed if malignancy is suspected but, in most cases, patients with recurrent oral ulceration should be screened for evidence of underlying or associated disease and can be treated satisfactorily only when this has been fully assessed and corrected where it exists. In patients with oral pain of non-dental origin, e.g. trigeminal neuralgia or tic douloureux, medical treatment with carbamazepine (Tegretol) is usually the treatment of choice but, if unsuccessful, surgical intervention may be required.

These examples illustrate the differences between the surgeon's and the physician's approach in the treatment of oral disease. In dentistry, these approaches may be successfully embodied in one individual but this book intends dealing with the physician's approach to oral health. The reader will often be aware of a lack of clear demarcation between oral surgery and oral medicine. This is to be expected and is consistent with the contemporary situation in general medicine where the dividing line between surgeon and physician is often indistinct and both may employ the same skills in diagnosis and treatment.

ORAL AND SYSTEMIC DISEASE

Disease of the body as a whole, systemic disease, often affects the mouth. Oral manifestations of systemic disease may be trivial and overshadowed by other ill effects of the systemic disorder or they may predate these other ill effects by weeks or months. Such oral manifestations may be confused with purely local diseases of the mouth and their prompt diagnosis by the dentist is essential. Oral medicine is that part of dentistry which is involved in the diagnosis and treatment of oral diseases of a non-surgical nature which may be localized to the mouth or which may be an oral manifestation of systemic disease.

Although oral medicine as defined above has been practised since the time of Hippocrates, its development has been slow when compared with that of oral surgery and oral pathology. The emergence of university departments of oral medicine in some dental schools reflects an increasing awareness of the systemic involvement in oral soft tissue disease and the need for special consideration in the management and treatment of such patients. Hitherto, patients with oral complaints such as dry mouth or recurrent ulceration have been treated by a variety of dental and medical specialists and by general practitioners. Patient care has depended on the traditional thinking and interests of the particular speciality to which the patient was referred, and co-ordination in the treatment of patients with oral soft tissue disease has often been lacking. Since it is also widely held that many disorders of the oral mucosa are troublesome but localized in nature and, in time, self-resolving, the consequent treatment has been empirical, non-specific and sometimes irrational, without consideration of the pathogenesis of the disorder being treated.

The general dental practitioner, by his training, experience and involvement in the regular review of his patients' mouths, is in a unique position to recognize early oral malignancy and oral signs of systemic disease. If advantage is to be taken of this by the profession, the practitioner must be backed by specialists in the field. These may practise only as oral physicians in large centres or may combine their practice of oral medicine with oral surgery.

In reviewing the interrelationship between oral and systemic disease it is important to consider whether oral disease can cause systemic abnormality. This is relevant since focal infection in the mouth is commonplace and any systemic ill effect of such infection would affect many members of the population. In the early years of this century the idea that focal sepsis caused systemic disease was promoted by Hunter, the famous British physician who described the glossitis associated with pernicious anaemia, and by others. In consequence, many patients had healthy as well as infected teeth extracted to prevent or treat diseases such as rheumatoid arthritis, iritis and dermatitis where the aetiology was unknown.

There is no evidence that dental or oral sepsis can cause these diseases and extractions of healthy teeth in these patients are not indicated. However, dental and periodontal infections can cause bacteraemia, and patients with congenital and rheumatic heart disease are at risk from subacute bacterial endocarditis as a result of this (see Chapter 9).

When a patient is referred by a doctor or physician for the elimination of focal sepsis the dentist should take a careful history and make a clinical examination with full mouth radiographs. In patients with congenital or rheumatic heart disease, the focal infection should be eliminated with appropriate antibiotic cover. A programme of long-term care should also be arranged to ensure that these patients do not develop chronic oral infections. In all other patients appropriate dental care, including root treatments, where necessary, will result in the elimination of foci of infection and indiscriminate and unhelpful extractions will be avoided.

THE ROLES OF DENTIST, DOCTOR AND HOSPITAL SPECIALIST

Patients suffering from dental decay almost invariably seek treatment from a dentist, but others suffering from oral complaints such as dryness or ulceration may visit either doctor or dentist and may be referred from one to the other because the dividing line between the professions of medicine and dentistry is not always clear. It follows that the family doctor (general medical practitioner), dentist (general dental practitioner) and specialists in various disciplines of dentistry and medicine may be concerned in the management of patients with oral disease. The purpose of this chapter is to consider the roles and interrelationship of these clinicians.

Until recently, general medical and dental practitioners usually practised separately and corresponded only occasionally by letter about certain patients and their care. Although the dental undergraduate receives basic instruction in the structure, function and diseases of the whole body, the information he acquires in these subjects may become stale through lack of opportunity to apply and develop it. Similarly, the medical student receives a little information in his undergraduate curriculum about teeth and the oral cavity in health or disease, but is provided with no practice in dentistry. However, it is gratifying that many medical and dental undergraduate curricula now contain the information necessary to enable doctors and dentists to provide complementary care for their patients. The advent of Health Centres or Primary Care Units in many countries has also encouraged liaison between doctors and dentists who may work in the same building, share the same supporting laboratory and ancillary services and jointly contribute to the total health care of their patients. It is often easier and more rewarding to discuss an unusual or complex patient management problem than to correspond about it and consultation occurs more easily when doctor and dentist work in the same clinical complex. The dentist should be aware of the need for consultation with the patient's doctor in some instances, and the doctor of complexities of dental care which fall outside his experience and training.

The hospital services of many countries produce excellent examples of co-operation between consultants and specialists in dentistry and medicine. The improved treatment of the cleft-palate patient is a good example of benefit derived from this team approach.

Failure of communication between doctor and dentist may be harmful, as in the following case. A patient presented to his general medical practitioner with facial pain and was prescribed an analgesic (aspirin) and a tranquillizer (diazepam). He was advised to consult his dentist to exclude a dental cause of facial pain. The dentist having found no dental cause diagnosed trigeminal neuralgia, prescribed dihydro-codeine and referred the patient to a consultant dental surgeon (specialist oral surgeon) who prescribed carbamazepine, which the patient took along with the dihydrocodeine, aspirin and diazepam. Obviously, such overprescribing is unnecessary and dangerous. Clearly one member of the health team should co-ordinate the drug treatment for a particular patient and, in the case described, the general medical practitioner was in the best position to co-ordinate treatment. The dentist and the consultant dental surgeon should have informed him and any medical specialist involved in the care of the patient of their findings and of any new treatment recommended by them. The dentist should not assume the role of a family doctor but should co-operate with the doctor in guarding the health and well-being of their joint patient.

REFERRAL OF PATIENTS

Requests for a specialist or consultant opinion may be made by a general medical practitioner or a general dental practitioner. In dentistry, the request may be for diagnosis, for treatment, or for advice regarding a plan of treatment which will be carried out by the general practitioner. The patient's well-being should always transcend personal pride and, in particular, a second opinion should be sought when the patient's complaint lies outside the practitioner's normal practice. When referring a patient, relevant information should be provided in advance and the consultant should reciprocate by letters to the general dental and medical practitioners when oral 'medical' disease is concerned.

A suitable outline for a referral letter is as follows:

(a) Name, address, telephone number and qualifications of referring practitioner.
(b) Name, address, age and sex of patient.
(c) Reason for referral. This should include a summary of the case history and the findings on clinical examination, the presumptive diagnosis and special note of any urgency. The practitioner should also indicate whether he wishes the specialist to undertake treatment or simply advise regarding treatment which the practitioner will provide.
(d) Information regarding present and recent drug therapy.
(e) Results of any special investigations recently undertaken. In particular, the practitioner may send relevant radiographs to avoid duplication and unnecessary radiation exposure.

THE ORAL MEDICINE CLINIC

It may be useful at this stage to consider the facilities which are available in some oral medicine clinics and the functions of these clinics. However, it should be recognized that in other centres such facilities may be provided in clinics dealing with oral surgery and oral medicine together or in joint medical and dental clinics. Clinics offering a specialist oral medicine service may be sited in general hospitals or in dental hospitals but in either instance they require the availability of radiological, microbiological, histopathological, biochemical, haematological and other specialist investigative services.

In practice, most patients attending an oral medicine clinic are referred from dental practitioners but referrals are made from most primary and specialist health areas. The patients come with a variety of complaints and it has been estimated that about one-quarter have underlying systemic disease which may cause their oral complaint.

Patients attending an oral medicine clinic require proper diagnosis. The method of diagnosis is detailed in Chapter 2. However, in the oral medicine clinic, facilities for full general, as well as intra-oral, examination are necessary. Side-rooms where patients with skin rashes or genital lesions can be examined should be available, and these side-rooms may be used for ancillary clinical tests. A small number of patients may require further in-patient investigation and beds should be available for oral medicine patients in medical wards. Facilities for joint consultation between the specialist in oral medicine and a dermatologist, or haematologist, psychiatrist or a general physician are often helpful and enable patient management and treatment to be provided with full appreciation of all the pertinent factors. Since the oral medicine clinic is involved in medical and dental matters it is also helpful to send reports in duplicate to medical and dental practitioners so that both may be informed of diagnosis, prognosis and treatment of patients with whom they may be concerned.

Special investigations form an important part of the work of an oral medicine clinic. The indications for special investigations are described throughout the text and the investigations used are summarized in Chapter 2 and in Appendix I. Here we are concerned with the general approach to these further tests. The student of oral medicine should be aware of the sampling techniques employed and the methods of general handling and transfer of materials to the laboratories. Haematological, biochemical, radiological and scintiscanning procedures may be required, and consultation with professional laboratory staff in pathology, microbiology, and in other disciplines may assist in diagnosis and point to further lines of investigation which may benefit the patient. In planning special investigations the clinician should consider the patient's contribution of time and effort. The investigations should entail a minimum of inconvenience. It is frustrating if several visits are required for investigation of patients when one co-ordinated investigative session would have sufficed.

An oral medicine clinic is staffed as is any other specialist clinic. The specialist (or consultant) oral physician is supported by junior staff who are often in training grades and are responsible for clerking and clinical examinations. Appropriate nursing, reception and secretarial assistance is also required. As indicated above, specialist physicians, dermatologists, haematologists, psychiatrists and rheumatologists may be in attendance at the clinic from time to time. Attendance at the oral medicine clinic is an important part of the dental undergraduate curriculum and may also benefit medical, nursing and other trainees. In this clinic, the dental student should study the normal appearance of the mouth, and its ecology and function. The methods of history-taking, clinical examination and diagnosis should be practised, and the student should acquire the ability to recognize common clinical signs such as ulceration, white lesions, bulla, inflammation and dryness. Students should be involved in the work of the clinic, taking case histories and elaborating programmes of investigation and diagnosis, under supervision. They should observe the treatment provided and the methods of referring patients between various specialist clinics. The medical undergraduate should be aware, too, of the range of dental and oral diseases and attendance at an oral medicine clinic may assist in achieving this end. In particular, he will have an opportunity of studying those oral diseases which are most likely to present in medical practice.

The oral medicine clinic provides helpful experience for other staff and postgraduate students training for hospital or academic careers in oral medicine or in oral surgery and also by doctors training in a variety of specialities. Tape/slide presentations for personal or small-group instruction is a most economical method of supplementing clinical experience and demonstrating the indications and techniques of special tests. In addition, dental ancillary staff and nurses should receive the widest possible training in all aspects of dentistry and this should include attendance at the oral medicine clinic. Dental ancillary workers such as hygienists should be aware of the appearance of disease of the oral mucosa so that they may report any abnormality to the dentist. Their routine duties include in-patient care in general hospitals where they must be conscious of the additional needs of certain patients; for example, those suffering from leukaemia.

Oral medicine clinics provide opportunities for research as well as for teaching. There is, for example, a need for an awareness of pharmacology and therapeutics in oral medicine; to this end, new drugs should be studied and evaluated. The clinic may be utilized to supervise clinical trials and to evaluate treatments for such conditions as recurrent aphthae, lichen planus and the oral bullous lesions. Clinical research today requires special biological techniques which demand considerable experience, and the use of sophisticated apparatus. For example, contemporary oral medicine research is involved with the biology of the cell in various disease states as assessed by electron microscopy, autoradiography and tissue culture. Of course, clinical research is undertaken with proper regard to ethical considerations and to the guidelines which exist in different countries for clinical research.

A. ADMISSION

TO BE COMPLETED WITHIN 14 DAYS OF FIRST ATTENDANCE AT THE DEPARTMENT

Card no. ☐ 1

Correction ☐ 2
(Enter 'X' only if this record has to overwrite a record on the master file — otherwise leave blank).

Sequence no. ☐☐☐☐☐ ☐ 3—8

Hospital no. ☐☐☐☐☐☐☐ 9—15

Surname ☐☐☐☐☐☐☐☐☐☐☐☐☐☐☐ 16—30

Initials ☐☐ 31—32

Date of birth ☐☐ ☐☐ ☐☐ 33—38

Sex ☐ 39
M. Male
F. Female

Race ☐ 40

Source of referral ☐ 41
1. Self
2. Gen. dental pract.
3. Gen. medical pract.
4. Special dental pract.
5. Special med. pract.
6. Other

Disposal ☐ 42
1. Discharge
2. Gen. dental pract.
3. Gen. medical pract.
4. Spec. dental pract.
5. Spec. med. pract.
6. Other

Pathology ☐ 43
1. Yes.
2. No.

Bacteriology ☐ 44
1. Yes.
2. No.

Category ☐ 45
1. Yes under-grad.
2. Yes post-grad.
3. Yes both.
4. No.

Suitable for clinical trial ☐ 46
1. Yes.
2. No.

Occupation ☐☐☐ 47—49

Date of presentation ☐☐ ☐☐ ☐☐ 50—55

Date of discharge ☐☐ ☐☐ ☐☐ 56—61

B. DIAGNOSIS

Card no. ☐ 1
(Enter '1' if site(s) relate to 1st diagnosis)
(Enter '2' if site(s) relate to 2nd diagnosis etc.)

Correction ☐ 2
(Enter 'X' only if this record has to overwrite a record on the Master File — otherwise leave blank)

Sequence no. ☐☐☐☐☐ ☐ 3—8

Hospital no. ☐☐☐☐☐☐☐ 9—15

Diagnosis ☐☐☐☐☐ 16—20

Sites ☐☐ 21—22 ☐☐ 23—24 ☐☐ 25—26 ☐☐ 27—28 ☐☐ 29—30

Figure 1.1. Information relating to patients attending the Department of Oral Medicine, Glasgow Dental Hospital.

Finally, in a discipline such as oral medicine, which involves the prolonged assessment of diseases and therapies, it is essential that clinical data should be readily available for statistical analysis for planning and research purposes. Various methods of card or computerized clinical and diagnostic abstracting may be used. Cases can be coded in accordance with the Dental Section of the *International Classification of Disease Index* (WHO document DH/69.83) with relevant patient and laboratory data. The correlation of clinical presentation with co-existent generalized disease states is now a simple operation, the reliability of which will increase with the progressive data input. When clinical trials are proposed, information can be obtained regarding patients who may be suitable for participation. A method of information coding for storage is shown in Figure 1.1. Two files of information are maintained, one of which contains individual patient data relevant to the case presentation. The other is a purely diagnostic file, one entry in which corresponds to one numerical ICD-DA code. This separation permits the rapid retrieval of information, either primarily patient orientated or diagnostically orientated. This simple method of computerized data storage may be the first stage of a more comprehensive system which could provide terminals within the clinic, giving instant access to information.

FURTHER READING

Mason, D. K., Chisholm, D. M., Ferguson, M. M., Hunter, I. P., Lyell, A. & Stephen, K. W. (1974) The function and organization of an oral medicine clinic. *British Dental Journal,* **136**, 460—466.

chapter 2

_____

Diagnosis and Treatment Planning

INTRODUCTION

Proper diagnosis requires more than knowledge of disease. It requires an ability to obtain information from patients by interview (the case history) and by physical examination. The information obtained is assessed against available knowledge of the presentation and behaviour of diseases to make a provisional or clinical diagnosis. The provisional diagnosis often points to further investigations which are aimed at reaching a final diagnosis. The treatment plan is based on the final diagnosis as is the prognosis or predicted outcome of the disease. These various stages are described in more detail in the sections which follow but description of them will be preceded by a brief consideration of the personal characteristics which patients exhibit and which are so important in determining the ease with which the facts may be obtained by the clinician. The clinician who hopes for a successful rapport with patients must also know the extent and limitations of his own knowledge, ability and personality.

It is not possible in this brief account to describe all the different physical and behavioural characteristics which patients may exhibit. A knowledge of these is built up slowly through experience and together with practice in diagnosis and an understanding of disease forms the basis of clinical wisdom. Thus, as the student studies disease processes in pathology every effort should be made to interview and examine as many patients as possible so that he may become an able diagnostician. Patients vary in age, experience, educational background and in many other ways.

Some are frightened, even to the extent of being unable to seek early help for their disorder. Others lack fear and may fail to show the usual response to certain situations. Some patients are anxious to assist but others appear unwilling to provide information as requested. Many patients hide essential facts in a mass of useless chatter and accounts of previous expert and inexpert diagnoses and treatments. Often, highly intelligent patients demand detailed explanations of their complaints while, in contrast, patients of low intelligence may respond only to simple explanations and questioning. Occasionally, patients are excessively demanding or difficult and then the clinician must remain calm and single-minded in order to achieve a proper diagnosis. The patient's well-being is always the desired endpoint and the clinician may vary the approach used in relation to the patient being interviewed.

The suggestion is made above that the clinician should also be aware of himself. In particular he should recognize personal limitations of knowledge or skill, particularly when he may be tired or ill, and the special restrictions of age. The careful clinician is quick to consult with colleagues when in doubt or if a patient's complaints fall outside his field of competence.

THE CASE HISTORY

The case history is based on an interview with the patient. It is a planned professional conversation which enables the patient to communicate his symptoms, feelings and fears to the clinician. From this information the clinician obtains insight into the nature of the patient's illness and his attitude to it.

The patient should be encouraged to tell his story voluntarily, the clinician only interrupting to obtain clarification of, or further information about, specific points. Often, however, patients are reluctant to speak freely and require some encouragement or a sympathetic response from the clinician. This may take the form of a visual or verbal expression of understanding. The least satisfactory case histories are those obtained by a series of questions from the clinician and monosyllabic answers from the patient. In such cases the clinician may be at fault in hurrying the procedure or in exhibiting impatience. Rarely, the patient lacks interest or the ability to describe symptoms and in these circumstances gentle questioning may be required.

A questionnaire which may serve as an aide-memoire and may be linked to a data analysis system suitable for card or computer systems is used by some clinicians. A disadvantage of this is the rigidity of the detail recorded: individual variations and the recording of events in sequence may be difficult to accommodate on questionnaires. While the history is being taken, the clinician should observe the patient's appearance, manner and reaction: is the reaction that expected of a patient with the complaint in question or is there an over-reaction with emotional or anxiety overtones, perhaps indicating the need of psychiatric assessment? Organic and psychiatric states may coexist and the one has an important bearing on the other. The case history should be recorded under the following headings:

(a) Personal data
(b) Present complaint(s)
(c) History and description of the present complaint(s)
(d) Previous history
(e) Social and family history

(a) **Personal data.** The personal data needed for the patient's record are usually collected by a receptionist but the clinician should be aware of this information. The patient's full name, address, telephone number, date of birth, sex, marital status, and occupation are usually listed, together with such reference numbers as are relevant to the clinician's institution or practice. The names, addresses and telephone numbers of other medical and dental attendants are useful on many occasions and reference numbers of other institutions relating to the patient may assist in obtaining relevant records about the case.

(b) **Present complaint(s).** These are best listed in simple terms in the order of priority given to them by the patient. For example, a patient may complain of:

(i)   Pain
(ii) Swelling
(iii) Bleeding gums
(iv) Bad breath

(c) **History and description of present complaint(s).** These should be recorded in the patient's own words, if possible. The history may concern a matter of hours or of several years and the events in it should be recorded chronologically. The patient should be questioned as to the precise meaning of the terms used. To the clinician, for instance, the term 'ulcer' implies a break or gap in the surface epithelium. The patient, in contrast, may use this term to describe an erythematous area which is not truly ulcerated. Patients usually wish to supply previous diagnoses of the condition; diagnoses which have been made by other clinicians or by relatives with no special knowledge of disease or training in medicine or dentistry. Such 'diagnoses' are rarely helpful and it is more important to obtain a catalogue of events and a description of symptoms in simple terms. An account of previous treatments is essential and may assist in diagnosis.

The clinician may supplement the patient's history and description of the present complaint by a series of questions. For example, if the patient has complained of pain the clinician must discover its site, nature, duration and whether any factors have aggravated or relieved it; also, whether the pain has radiated to other parts of the body or has occurred previously.

(d) **Previous history.** This incorporates a general medical history and a dental history. To begin with, the patient may be asked three general questions: Are you completely well at present? Have you suffered any serious illness or had any major surgical operation in the past? Do you have any complaints at present, other than those relating to your mouth which you have already spoken of? These questions should be followed by another series, designed to ascertain any evidence of major disease of parts of the body other than the mouth. The patient who admits to dyspnoea, chronic cough, chest pain or peripheral oedema may suffer from disease of the cardiorespiratory systems. All patients should be asked whether they have suffered from rheumatic fever, chorea, valvular heart disease, other heart disease, or lung disease. Vomiting, acid regurgitation, abdominal pain or alteration in bowel habit may indicate disease of the gastrointestinal tract. Patients should also be questioned about previous jaundice and liver disease. Other important symptoms which may indicate internal disease include weight loss; bleeding with the appearance of blood in the sputum, vomitus, urine, or faeces; and unexplained pain. Women of childbearing age should be asked if they are pregnant, particularly if radiographs are to be taken. Special note should be made of diabetes, thyroid and other endocrine disorders. Patients should be asked if they have had any skin diseases or arthritis. A history of psychiatric disorder or other disease of the nervous system may be relevant.

It is important that present and recent drug therapy be recorded and patients must be questioned about possible allergy to drugs or to other agents. The clinician must be aware, also, of any tendency to bleeding or bruising exhibited by the patient and of any previous episode of excessive bleeding following trauma or surgery.

The previous history in patients with oral disease should include a reference to the dental history. Regularity of attendance, date of last treatment and the name of the practitioner providing it, types of dental treatment received in the past and complications such as bleeding or reaction to local anaesthetic should all be ascertained.

(e) **Social and family history.** This should include queries about occupation and hobbies. Habits in respect of tobacco and alcohol usage may be important in certain diseases. Family illnesses may be relevant and where a history of the patient's complaint is uncovered in relatives it may be helpful to record a 'family tree' which should indicate those members of the family affected by the disease.

PHYSICAL EXAMINATION OF THE PATIENT

The patient should be examined thoroughly. Obviously, the dental situation restricts the examination to those parts of the body which are readily visible. The following section deals with this type of procedure. A more complete examination is possible in medical practice but the physician may lack the expertise, equipment, or lighting to examine all parts of the mouth. Nevertheless, the restricted examination which is carried out by the dentist may yield important clues in the diagnosis of internal disease, and much can be discovered in the mouth with little more than good lighting and the simplest spatula.

The clinician should observe the patient from the moment he enters the clinic, noting his walk, posture, and general appearance and attitude. These characteristics alter with age but the experienced clinician will identify some patients as 'ill' as they enter. The clinician should study the character and colour of the skin; the general facial expression which may suggest anxiety or other emotional state; the conjunctivae which may reveal pigmentation as in jaundice; and the general form of the face with particular reference to facial asymmetry and swelling. The cervical glands on both sides should be palpated from behind; after the shirt collar has been unbuttoned, in a man's case. Other lymphatic glands in axilla and groin may require examination. The salivary glands should be palpated and bimanual palpation of the submandibular glands is necessary. Examples of the methods of extra-oral examination are illustrated in Figure 2.1. Some of the abnormalities which can be observed from extra-oral examination are shown in Figure 2.2(a—d).

Intra-orally, the lips, buccal mucosa, oropharynx, tongue (dorsal and ventral surface and lateral margins), floor of mouth, palate and gingiva should be examined in sequence. Complete visualization with good light is essential. The buccal mucosa should be extended laterally and the tongue should be protruded, the tip held by the examiner using a linen gauze strip in order to expose dorsal and ventral surfaces, the lateral border, and foliate and circumvallate papillae. The location, appearance, size, colour and distribution of any lesions present should be recorded. The appearance of the normal oral mucosa at different sites is shown in Figure 2.3 (a—f) and examples of common abnormalities are shown in Figure 2.4(a—d).

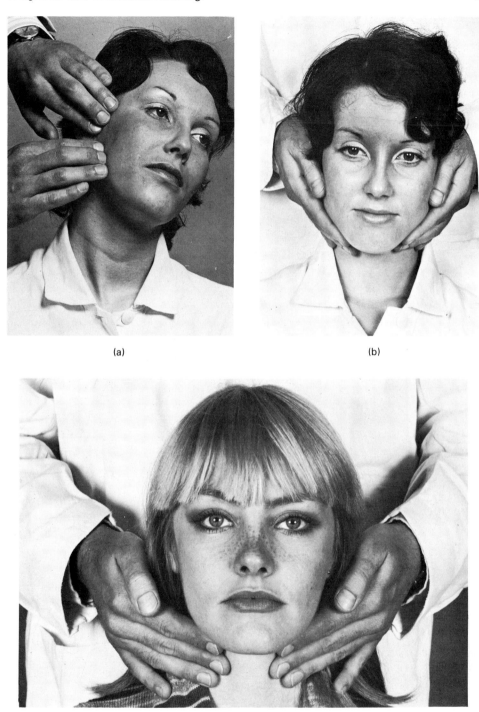

(a)   (b)

(c)

Figure 2.1. Bimanual palpation of (a) the parotid gland region, (b) the right and left submandibular gland region, and (c) the neck.

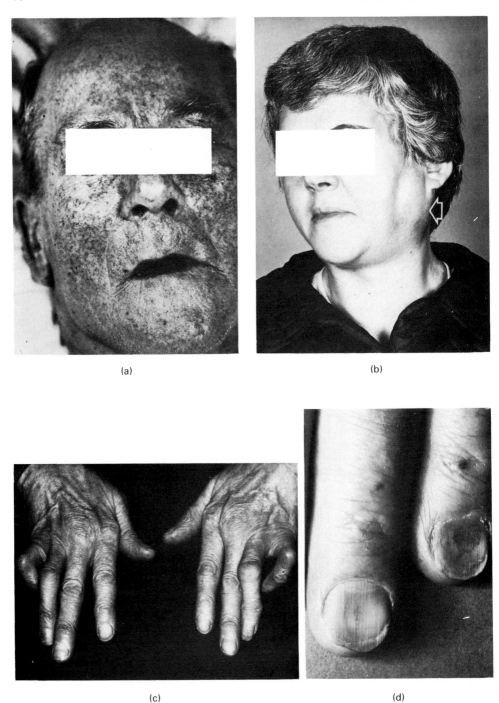

(a)

(b)

(c)

(d)

Figure 2.2. (a) 'Spider naevi' in a patient with liver disease; (b) swelling of the left parotid gland (arrowed) in a patient with Sjögren's syndrome; (c) involvement of the metacarpal-phalangeal joints in a case of rheumatoid arthritis; and (d) longitudinal striations on the finger nails in a case of lichen planus.

The teeth present should be recorded and then examined for any morphological or structural abnormalities such as hypoplasia, staining and caries. The gums should be examined for gingivitis and periodontal disease, and the form of the occlusion should be recorded with special reference to any mal-relation of the teeth or malocclusion (Figure 2.5).

A number of special clinical terms are used to describe oral mucosal appearances and these are defined below and illustrated diagrammatically in Figure 2.6.

Macule: a circumscribed non-raised area of altered coloration varying in size from pinhead to several centimetres. It is usually deeper in colour than the surrounding tissue. Petechiae, the tiny haemorrhages seen in scurvy or thrombocytopenic purpura and melanin deposits as in Addison's disease, are examples of macules.

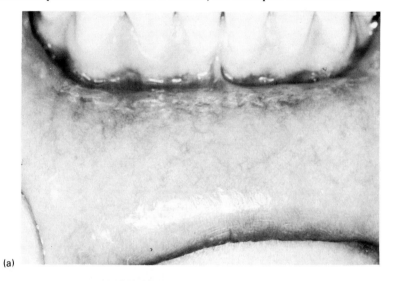

(a)

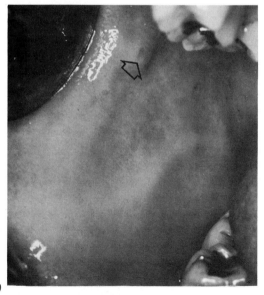

(b)

Figure 2.3. Normal appearance of the oral mucosa at the following sites: (a) lower lip; (b) cheek (parotid duct orifice indicated).

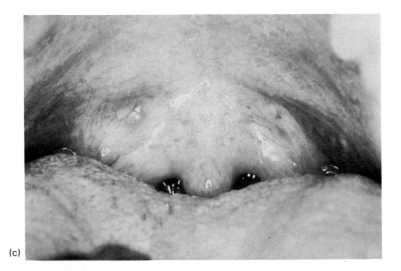

(c)

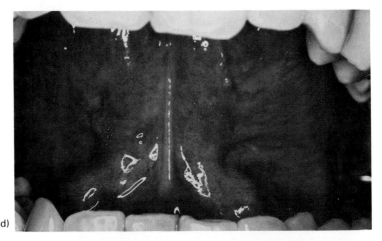

(d)

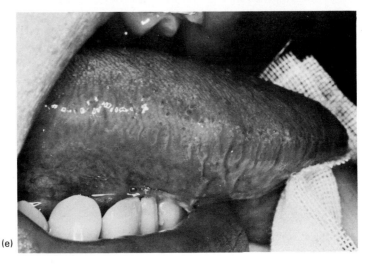

(e)

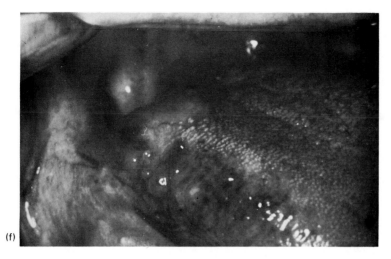

(f)

Figure 2.3. Normal appearance of the oral mucosa at the following sites: (c) soft palate; (d) undersurface of tongue; (e) lateral border of tongue; and (f) circumvallate papilla.

Papule: a small circumscribed elevated area, with a round or ovoid base. The surface may be rounded, flattened or pointed. Usually oral papules are grey/white in colour. Lichen planus is an example of a disease in which papules may appear.

Plaque: a slightly raised clearly demarcated area of grey or white coloration. The surface may be smooth or pebbled and cracks or fissures may be seen dividing the lesion. Leukoplakia, carcinoma and discoid lupus erythematosus are examples of diseases which may appear as plaques.

Vesicle: a small circumscribed elevated blister, not more than 5 mm in diameter, with a thin covering layer of epithelial cells and containing an accumulation of fluid. Vesicles can be single or multiple and they appear in varying stages of formation and healing. The covering membrane may be thick, as in a subepithelial vesicle, or thin when intra-epithelial. As the vesicular membrane ruptures an ulcer is formed. Examples are burns and herpetic lesions of the mucous membranes.

Bulla: similar to a vesicle, although generally the term is restricted to lesions larger than 5 mm in diameter. Again the covering epithelium may be thick or thin depending on whether the bulla is intra-epithelial or subepithelial. Pemphigus and pemphigoid are diseases characterized by bulla formation.

Pustule: a vesicular type of lesion which contains pus within the cavity of the vesicle.

Ulcer: a break or discontinuity in the surface epithelium of the skin or mucous membrane. The floor of the ulcer consists of connective tissue which is covered by a fibrinous exudate infiltrated by polymorphs. Ulcers differ in type: they may have 'punched-out' edges, as in aphthae; 'undermined' edges, as in tuberculosis; or 'raised' or 'rolled' edges, as in malignancy.

Erosion: a shallow defect in the oral mucosa representing a loss of epithelium down to and sometimes including the stratum germinativum but without any loss of deeper structures. Erosions occur in some forms of lichen planus.

Nodule: a circumscribed condensation of tissue which may project from the surface as a polyp. It usually consists of fibrous tissue with an epithelial covering. Fibrous overgrowths are common examples.

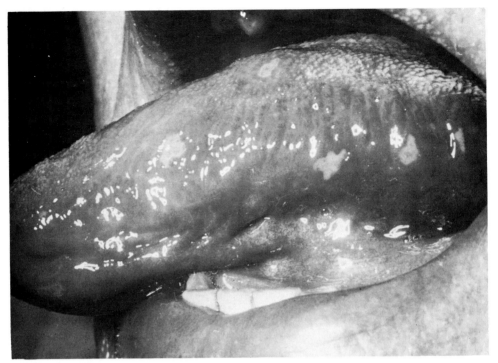

(a)

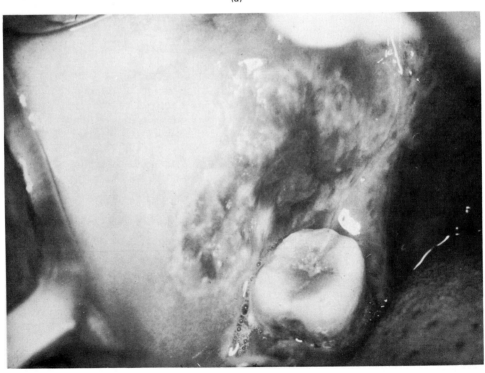

(b)

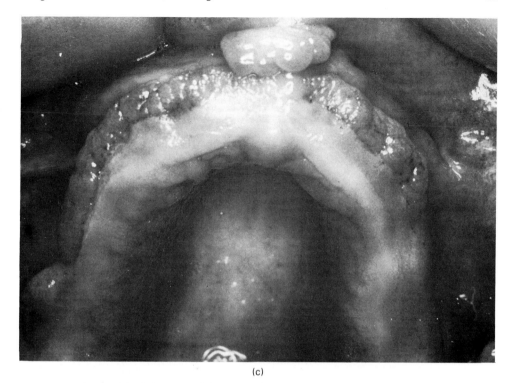

(c)

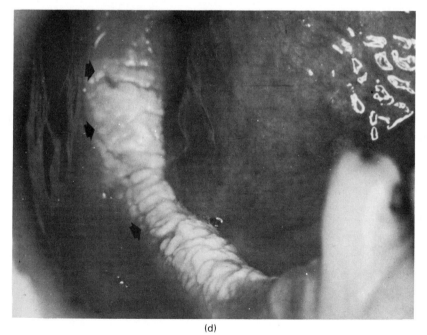

(d)

Figure 2.4. Abnormalities of the oral mucosa: (a) aphthous ulcers on lateral border of tongue; (b) lichen planus of buccal mucosa; (c) denture-induced hyperplasia of maxillary alveolar mucosa; and (d) leukoplakia of R. mandibular alveolar mucosa.

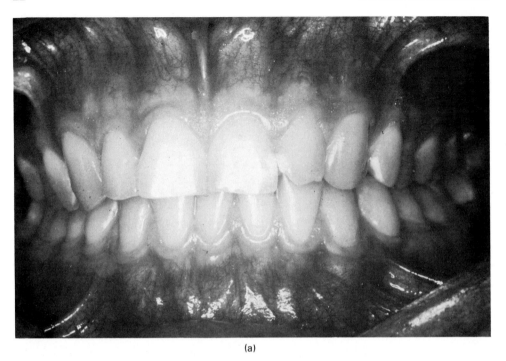

(a)

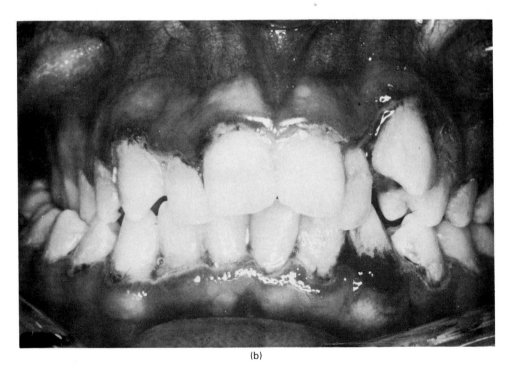

(b)

Figure 2.5. Contrast between (a) healthy teeth and good occlusion and (b) severe malocclusion and extensive periodontal disease.

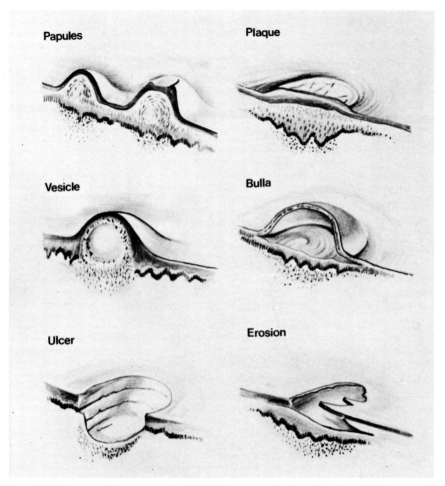

Figure 2.6. Diagrammatic representation of clinical terms used to describe oral mucosal appearances.

Atrophy: the term implies a shrinkage or reduction in size of an organ or part. Atrophy of the mucous membrane produces a thin red appearance. The smooth red surface on the dorsum of the tongue in iron deficiency is an example. It is important that the redness associated with mucosal atrophy be differentiated from that found in erythroplasia.

THE PROVISIONAL DIAGNOSIS

On completion of the case history and the physical examination, the clinician must determine what disease (or diseases) are likely to present with the symptoms and signs exhibited by the patient. At this stage the diagnosis may be imprecise and the clinician may be unable to decide which of several diseases is at fault. For example, a patient's oral ulceration may be a manifestation of many diseases including infections, recurrent aphthae, nutritional deficiencies, bullous disorders, trauma, leukaemia, ulcerative colitis, drug ingestion and tumours. The critical points in the case history and physical examination would include sites involved, duration (intermittent or recurrent), pain, sequence leading to ulceration (e.g., preceding vesicles or bullae), general health, skin lesions, alimentary symptoms and medication.

The clinician might suspect the final diagnosis from careful assessment of the available data but confirmation of this diagnosis would almost certainly require further investigation. Such investigations are outlined in the sections which follow. Making a provisional diagnosis may be time-consuming but it is an important stage in reaching a final diagnosis, and investigations carried out without regard to the clinical data already available may lead the clinician astray.

INVESTIGATIONS

A wide variety of investigations is available. Those most frequently utilized in oral medicine are: (a) radiology; (b) haematology; (c) biochemistry; (d) immunology; (e) microbiology; (f) histopathology.

Other specialized tests may be used, for example those of salivary gland function, which include: (a) flow rate studies; (b) biopsy; (c) sialography; (d) scintiscanning.

It is important that the patient be informed of the reason for special tests and further investigations, and when several are required these should be planned carefully in order to minimize inconvenience to the patient.

Details of the methods relating to these tests are contained in Appendix I at the end of this book and indications for their use are described in various chapters throughout the text. However, some of the tests listed above require the removal of tissue, blood or saliva for examination. Methods used in these will now be described.

Biopsy

The taking of a biopsy specimen is an important though relatively simple procedure. Selection of the site entails choosing a representative area of the lesion in question. The most accurate method of removing tissue for biopsy specimen is the incisional method. A small lesion, however, may be completely removed and the technique in this case is known as excisional biopsy. Prior to biopsy, anaesthesia is obtained by block injection or local infiltration around the lesion but not into the site itself. Using a scalpel, an elliptical or V-shaped incision is made. It should include the periphery of the lesion and be deep enough so that appropriate pathologically altered tissue is present. The specimen should be dissected away and removed gently, care being taken not to tear or distort the tissue. Bleeding is controlled by gauze and pressure. A few fine black silk sutures may be required to close the wound. The specimen is mounted on a small piece of blotting paper and immersed immediately in a fixative, usually 10 per cent formaldehyde solution. The incisional biopsy technique is shown in Figure 2.7(a—c). In submitting a biopsy specimen to the pathologist, the clinician should ensure that all details on the histopathology request form are completed.

Punch biopsy may be used to obtain tissue from an inaccessible area, or where incisional biopsy is not practical or when multiple samples from an extensive lesion are required. For this, a special instrument which removes a small fragment or core of tissue is employed. Oral exfoliative cytology may be used to complement these biopsy techniques.

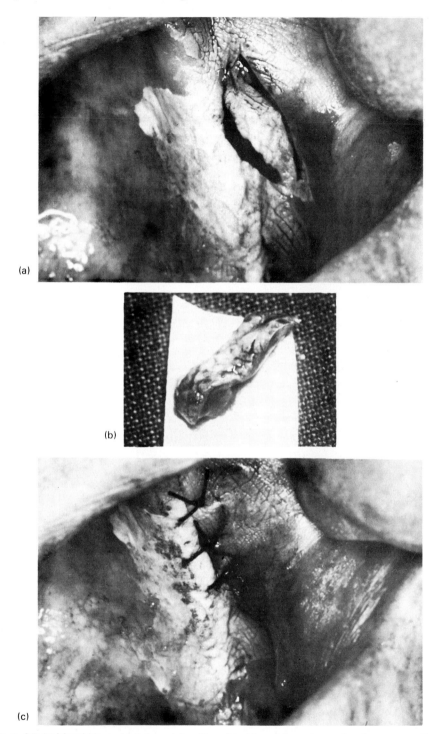

(a)

(b)

(c)

Figure 2.7. Incisional biopsy technique: (a) outline of incision; (b) specimen placed upon a small piece of blotting paper; and (c) wound closed with black silk sutures. The white patch lesion affects the upper left alveolar ridge and cheek.

The Collection of Venous Blood for Analysis

Blood may be conveniently collected from the arm veins in the antecubital fossa.

A small tray should be available with all the necessary equipment, including the specimen bottles, but the equipment, especially the syringe needle, should be kept out of sight until it is to be used. The patient should be asked to expose the forearm and upper arm above the antecubital fossa. A tourniquet is gently applied around the upper arm and the cephalic and basilic veins should be visualized or palpated. A co-operative patient may occlude the veins by gripping the upper arm with the free hand, but in most cases it is best to use an elastic strip (proprietary), rubber tube or sphygmomanometer cuff. If the veins do not distend after the tourniquet is applied, the patient should open and close the hand to increase the venous pressure. This procedure should be used only when necessary as it can alter the concentration of certain blood chemical constituents, such as serum potassium.

Before the needle is inserted, the skin is prepared by washing with a surface solution, e.g. 5 per cent chlorhexidine in 70 per cent alcohol. The needle is inserted obliquely through the skin in the line of the vein (Figure 2.8). Resistance is encountered when the

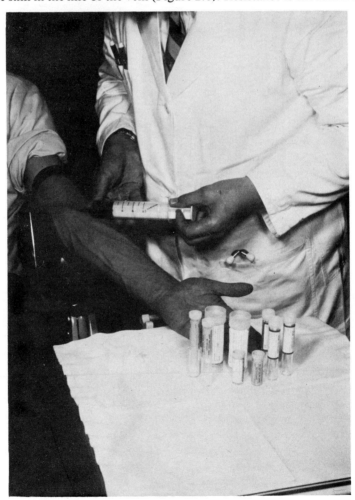

Figure 2.8. Removal of venous blood.

needle meets the vein wall. This is overcome when the wall is perforated and the needle comes to lie in the vein lumen. The venous blood is withdrawn slowly and when sufficient has been obtained the tourniquet is removed, a gauze swab is placed over the needle insertion site and the needle and syringe are removed. The patient is asked to hold the swab over the skin puncture site and the arm is raised above the level of the heart. The needle should be removed from the syringe and the blood expressed from the syringe into the specimen tube (Figure 2.9). Care should be taken to avoid spillage of blood or contamination of the hands of operator or assistants with blood. Where the patient is jaundiced or gives a history of jaundice, gloves should be worn, and the specimen specially labelled so that the laboratory staff may take suitable precautions. These steps are intended to avoid the risk of serum hepatitis and, after use, needles and syringes should be disposed of properly.

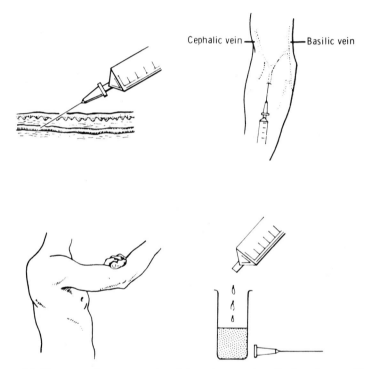

Figure 2.9. Diagrammatic representation of the main stages in collection of venous blood.

   Venous blood can be obtained simply from most patients, but there are certain patients with whom difficulties may be encountered, and in cases such as the following there is no substitute for experience:

1. In the older patient with sclerotic veins and thin connective tissues, it may be necessary to steady the vein with one hand in order to prevent it moving when the needle meets its thickened wall. Alternatively, a vein fixed by a Y-junction can be used.
2. In the fat patient, veins may be difficult to visualize. The tourniquet should not be applied too tightly and it may be helpful to palpate the vein before inserting the needle.

The Collection of Saliva for Analysis

Saliva to determine salivary flow rate or for the estimation of a biochemical constituent may be collected as mixed saliva or as separated gland secretions from parotid, submandibular, sublingual or minor glands. In clinical practice, mixed saliva or parotid saliva is usually collected by the spitting or drainage methods.

Spitting Method

The subject is seated with the head inclined forward so that the saliva will collect anteriorly in the floor of the mouth. He then spits the saliva thus produced into a collecting filter funnel once every minute for a given time, the length of which depends on the purpose of the investigation. A bench clock with a minute hand should be placed in front of the subject in order that the spitting procedure can be self-regulated.

Drainage Method

The subject is seated with the head inclined forwards so that the saliva produced will collect anteriorly in the floor of the mouth and flow out over the lip. The saliva is collected in a funnel connected to graduated measuring tubes. Before starting the collection, the subject should swallow all the saliva present in his mouth. At the end, all the saliva remaining in the mouth should be ejected into the container to ensure that the viscous minor gland secretion is also obtained.

Stimulated mixed saliva may be obtained by getting the patient to chew some inert material such as rubber bands.

Parotid saliva is best collected using a modified Carlson—Crittenden cup. This is a two-chambered device which is held in position over the parotid duct orifice by air suction applied through the outer chamber. The saliva flows through the inner chamber along a tube to the collection tube. It is important to decide whether the saliva will be collected under 'resting' conditions or when using a stimulus. Stimulated saliva is usually chosen, particularly when the secreting capacity of a gland is to be assessed. The flow rate should be determined when assessing the salivary concentration of a particular constituent because wide variations can occur at different flow rates. In addition, such factors as age, sex, plasma level, diurnal variation, drug therapy, and duration and type of stimulus have to be considered in relation to the parameter being measured.

A suitable clinical test using 10 per cent citric acid as a stimulus is as follows:

1. The subject is seated comfortably in a dental chair and the procedure is explained.
2. The collection device is fitted (Figure 2.10). Five drops of 10 per cent citric acid solution are dropped on the tongue from a 10 ml disposable syringe to flush out stagnant secretions for 15 minutes and to avoid rest transients.
3. Saliva is collected (Figure 2.11) under 'resting' conditions for 30 minutes, and after 10 per cent citric acid stimulation for two minutes. The citric acid is applied for at least one minute before the collection of the stimulated sample.

In clinical practice, the rate of flow is usually obtained by dividing the volume of saliva secreted in unit time by the duration of the collection period. Using this method, normal values for resting and stimulated saliva have been defined (Table 2.1). Details of techniques for saliva collection from different glands, the measurement of salivary flow rate and the normal ranges of salivary constituents are available in standard textbooks on the subject.

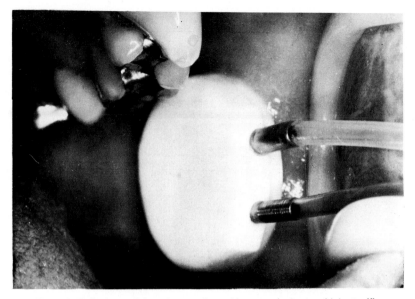

Figure 2.10. Carlson — Crittenden cup, in position over the L. parotid duct orifice.

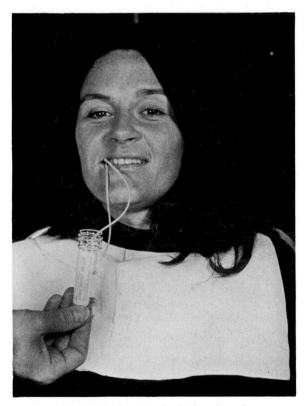

Figure 2.11. Parotid saliva being collected.

Table 2.1. *Mean parotid salivary flow rates in normal subjects (ml/min).*

Age range (years)		Resting		Fruit gum		Lemon juice	
		Male	Female	Male	Female	Male	Female
<20	18 M	0.061±0.007 (0.02−0.12)		0.66±0.06 (0.36−1.07)		1.49±0.09 (0.60−2.10)	
	8 F		0.083±0.02 (0.04−0.16)		0.46±0.07 (0.27−0.80)		1.99±0.14 (1.25−2.50)
21−40	20 M	0.104±0.008 (0.06−0.20)		0.47±0.03 (0.32−0.85)		1.73±0.09 (0.85−2.99)	
	20 F		0.09±0.01 (0.01−0.19)		0.50±0.05 (0.09−1.04)		1.76±0.09 (1.03−2.70)
41−60	27 M	0.078±0.02 (0.01−0.31)		0.59±0.08 (0.15±1.76)		1.68±0.11 (0.85−3.20)	
	31 F		0.064±0.01 (0.01−0.34)		0.52±0.05 (0.13−1.15)		1.36±0.12 (0.50−3.02)
>61	14 M	0.084±0.02 (0.03±0.20)		0.050±0.08 (0.15−1.26)		1.58±0.16 (0.90−2.76)	
	31 F		0.06±0.02 (0.01−0.5)		0.43±0.03 (0.14−0.83)		1.15±0.08 (0.47−2.20)

Mean ± Standard error of the mean (S.E.M.). Ranges indicated in parenthesis.
From Mason and Chisholm (1975).

THE FINAL DIAGNOSIS

A further review of the case is made after completion of the planned investigations. A final diagnosis is made. Not infrequently, several diseases have been identified and these should be listed, giving priority to that causing the patient's original complaint, unless a more serious disease has been discovered during the procedures outlined above. The patient and others concerned with his health care should be informed of the final diagnosis, an example of which is given here:

1. Leukoplakia tongue and palate.
2. Caries, listing the affected teeth.
3. Chronic marginal gingivitis.
4. Microcytic anaemia with iron deficiency.

TREATMENT PLANNING

The clinician should formulate a treatment plan based on the final diagnosis. Treatment should be provided with regard to the patient's convenience; visits to hospitals and clinics should be planned with this end in view. The treatment plan should be discussed with the patient and his consent to it obtained. Again, others concerned with the patient's health care should be informed of the treatment plan and this opportunity is usually taken to tell them of the main findings in respect of the case and of the prognosis.

A possible treatment plan in respect of the diagnosis given above is as follows:

1. Excise leukoplakic area of tongue.
2. Observe leukoplakia elsewhere in the mouth at three-monthly intervals.
3. Advise against possible local irritants such as cigarette smoking.
4. Refer to dentist for treatment of caries and periodontitis.
5. Refer to physician for investigation and treatment of anaemia.

THE PROGNOSIS

Proper treatment planning requires an assessment of the likely outcome of the diseases which have been identified. Precise prognosis is often impossible or can be given only as a statistic. For example, it may be known that one patient in 10 of those who suffer from the disease in question will develop a squamous carcinoma within five years. Obviously, this knowledge will influence the advice given to the patient and, perhaps, his willingness to take that advice. The patient must not be threatened by the possible consequences of the disease to the extent that anxiety results. Words such as cancer and malignancy should not be used. Nevertheless, he should be informed in simple terms that the treatment plan outlined by the clinician is necessary. Questions should be answered simply, with regard to the patient's character and personality. A positive hopeful approach with emphasis on the steps to be taken is best and the patient should be encouraged to join with the clinician in completing the treatment plan. Some aspects of treatment are wholly in his own hands; for example, following the advice which may be given in respect of cigarette smoking and other habits. If the disease in question is not malignant, the patient must be reassured and an opportunity given to him for voicing fears regarding cancer and death which he may not have mentioned at an earlier stage. The patient should be reassured gently and firmly in respect of such fears. Where a more serious disease is present, consultation with the physician should precede disclosure of the diagnosis so that full regard can be taken of the patient's personality, background and of the support which is to be provided. In such circumstances, the emphasis is always on the hopeful aspects of the treatment which is to be provided. The clinician should avoid holding conversations with colleagues, ancillary staff or students within sight of the patient. These might be construed by the patient as referring to his case and describing some dire consequence of his disease. Such conversations have often caused needless anxiety to patients and, as always, all activity in the clinic should be patient-orientated.

CONCLUSIONS

The description of the method of diagnosis and treatment planning given above is necessarily brief. It cannot be emphasized too strongly that practice in diagnosis is more important than reading about it.

An example of the stages in case-history taking, and the management of the patient from initial presentation or referral to the final diagnosis and prognosis, will now be given:

APPENDIX: EXAMPLE OF MANAGEMENT OF A CLINICAL CASE

Details	Comments
1. Personal Details	
NAME: Jean Smith Unit no: 654321 Date of Birth: 19 October 1910 Sex: F. Marital Status: Widow Race: Caucasian. Occupation: Dancer (ret.) Address: 12 Any Road, New Town GDP: Mr I. Pullit, New Town GMP: Dr P. Green, New Town	Before the clinician meets the patient he should review the information available to him. This includes the personal details of the patient as well as the letter of referral (if any).
2. Case History	
(a) Complaints:	

(i)   Oral ulceration.
    (ii) Cracks at corners of mouth.
    (iii) Pain on ridge in /5 region.
	Complaints are listed in order to facilitate a full diagnosis and treatment plan. If these are not specifically listed, features tend to be obscured in a long or complex history.

(b) History of Present Conditions:	
(i) Ulcers: started 6 months ago and occur on buccal and labial mucosae, as well as on soft palate. Usual size is about 5 mm and these last for 7—10 days. Severity is possibly increasing. No such previous history. No other skin or mucosal ulceration (i.e., nose, eyes, vaginal, perianal).	Ulcers sound like recurrent aphthae, with typical mucosal distribution. Unusual feature is late onset in this patient. Patient is sure that blisters do not develop prior to ulceration and there is no involvement of other mucosal surfaces or skin to suggest bullous disorder.

Details	Comments
(ii) Cracks at corners of mouth: these have been troublesome for at least 5 years, and the cracks tend to come and go. In the past 6 months, the cracks have been persistent.	Several aetiological factors might be associated with angular cheilitis. At this stage consideration should be made of a single cause for oral ulceration and angular cheilitis, e.g., nutritional deficiency.
(iii) Pain on ridge in $/5$ region: present for 5—10 years and is particularly troublesome if she wears lower denture. Pain is not severe, but she now leaves lower denture out for much of the time. Pain does not radiate.	Would appear to be local problem and sounds either as if denture is causing pressure on a lesion in the ridge or the denture itself is traumatizing the ridge. Could the absence of lower denture be a factor causing angular cheilitis?

(c) Dental History:

Teeth removed 25 years ago. Present dentures 12 years old. Never any problems with local anaesthetics or post-extraction haemorrhage.	No obvious problem. Present dentures are now fairly old.

(d) Medical History:

Myocardial infarction 8 years ago. Being treated for hypertension (mild). No history of respiratory disease, allergy, jaundice or rheumatic fever. Diet adequate. Weight possibly decreased in recent months. Bowel habits are presently a bit irregular. No haemorrhoids that she knows of.	Reasonable history for 67-year-old individual. Alimentary symptoms are a bit vague, but these may be relevant.

(e) Drugs:

Thiazide diuretic for hypertension.	This should not cause any of her presenting problems.

(f) Social History:

Lives with daughter. Smokes 20 cigarettes per day. Alcohol occasionally.	Nothing significant.

(g) Family History:

No known F.H. of oral ulceration. Eldest of 3 sisters — others alive and well. One parent died from cerebral thrombosis and the other from abdominal carcinoma.	Nothing apparently significant.

3. Clinical Examination

(a) Extra-oral:

Fit looking lady. No facial swelling or asymmetry. Bilateral angular cheilitis with crusting. No cervical lymphadenopathy. No rash on visible skin.	General observations and extra-oral examination reveal only angular cheilitis.

(b) Intra-oral

Edentulous — wearing upper complete denture. Oral mucosa is moist and saliva is flowing from all 4 major salivary gland duct orifices. Two ulcers present on right buccal mucosa and one on lower labial mucosa: all 5 mm in diameter and appear like aphthae. Spicule of calcified material projecting through mucosa on ridge in $/5$ region. Hard palate appears erythematous under upper denture, which is not well retained.	Intra-oral examination reveals ulcers which are consistent with recurrent aphthae. Lesion on lower ridge may be a fragment of a root or bony spicule projecting through mucosa. Palate has the appearance of denture stomatitis and, regardless of lesion on ridge, dentures are probably inadequate.

Details	**Comments**

4. Provisional Diagnosis

    (i)   Recurrent aphthae of recent onset.
    (ii) Angular cheilitis.
    (iii) Root or alveolar bone projecting through on lower ridge, $\overline{5}$ region.
    (iv) Denture stomatitis.

Several diagnoses which, although having separate elements, could overlap in aetiology, or provoking factors. Further investigations will be required.

5. Further Investigations

(a) For ulcers: Hb, MCV (mean corpuscular volume), MCH (mean corpuscular haemoglobin).
Serum iron and TIBC (total iron binding capacity).
Serum ferritin.
Corrected Whole Blood Folate.
Serum vitamin B_{12}.

Investigations designed to detect nutritional deficiency which could be causing oral ulceration.

(b) For Angular cheilitis:

Smears and swabs from both angles for bacteriology.
Swab from nose to detect possible *Staph.* source.
Smears and swabs from denture (see below).
Haematological investigations as for ulcers.

Several organisms can be involved in secondary infection in angular cheilitis.
Reservoir for *Staph. aureus* can be nose and candida may be mouth.
Nutritional deficiency can also cause angular cheilitis.

(c) Lesion on lower ridge:

Periapical radiograph of $\overline{5}$ region and orthopantomogram (OPT).

Radiography of lesion to reveal nature of calcified mass. OPT as a method of surveying remainder of ridges for a similar problem elsewhere.

(d) Denture Stomatitis:

Smears and swabs from the fitting surface of upper denture and from hard palate.

Candida is more often found on denture surface in cases of denture stomatitis. Smears will reveal candida in hyphal (i.e., pathological) phase of growth.

6. Results of Investigations

(a) Hb 12.2 g/dl. MCV 81 fl (81 μ^3). Blood film normal. Serum iron 5 μmol/l. TIBC 62 μmol/l (saturation 8.1 per cent). Serum ferritin 6. Folate and B_{12} normal.

Although the peripheral blood appears normal there is clear evidence of iron deficiency (saturation <16 per cent).

(b) Bacteriology reports *Staphylococcus aureus* and *Candida albicans* isolated from both angles. No *Staph.* from nose. *Candida albicans* from denture and palate.

Mixed infections in angular cheilitis are common. Reservoir of candida in mouth must be considered.

(c) Radiograph shows root fragment on ridge in $\overline{5}$ area. Alveolar bone otherwise normal.

Simple local lesion.

(d) Bacteriology report from denture and palate shows *Candida albicans* in hyphal phase.

Consistent with diagnosis of denture stomatitis.

7. Provisional Treatment Plan

(a) Determine cause of iron deficiency. Consultation with general physician: in view of good dietary history and no obvious blood loss, as well as vague alimentary symptoms, general examination, faecal occult blood, barium meal and barium enema.

Cause of iron deficiency *must* be established. The general investigations are conducted in a sequence as indicated. In view of other therapy — no local treatment given for aphthae. If there had been no intra-oral candida then a chlorhexidine mouthwash would have been prescribed at this stage.

Details	Comments

(b) Clear secondary infection from angles with miconazole cream.

Miconazole is active against candida as well as staphylococci.

(c) Remove root from ridge in /5 region.

Simple procedure.

(d) Treat denture stomatitis with amphotericin lozenges as well as applying amphotericin cream to fitting surface of upper denture.

This should produce response fairly rapidly and permit impressions to be taken. Approach may have to be adapted according to severity.

(e) Arrange to have new dentures constructed, ensuring that vertical dimension and anterior component are satisfactory.

Old dentures were inadequate. Adequate vertical dimension assists in controlling angular cheilitis.

8. Final Diagnosis and Response to Treatment

(a) General investigation revealed an early carcinoma in descending colon which was bleeding into lumen. This was at an early stage and was resected. Patient made a good recovery.
Oral iron was given for three months in order to restore tissue stores.
Oral ulceration cleared completely, one month after operation.

Iron deficiency was presumably due to blood loss from carcinoma. This was of fairly short duration and explains recent onset of aphthae. Also emphasizes need to measure iron directly rather than depend upon haemoglobin.

(b) Angular cheilitis cleared with regular use of miconazole and provision of new dentures.

Aetiology of angular cheilitis was probably due to loss of vertical dimension from not wearing lower denture. However, the recent deterioration may well have been caused by the iron deficiency.

(c) Root was removed from /5 region and wound healed.

(d) Denture stomatitis improved, permitting impressions to be taken.

(e) New upper and lower dentures constructed, which patient found acceptable.

FURTHER READING

Kerr, D. A., Ash, M. N. & Millard, H. D. (1978) *Oral Diagnosis.* St Louis, U.S.A.: Mosby.
Mason, D. K. & Chisholm, D. M. (1975) *Salivary Glands in Health and Disease.* London, Philadelphia, Toronto: W. B. Saunders.

part 2

DISEASE OF THE
ORAL MUCOSA

chapter *3*

Development, Structure and Disorders of Development

Development
Structure
Disorders of Development
Miscellaneous Lesions

DEVELOPMENT

By the third week of fetal life, the primitive mouth cavity (stomatodaeum) is formed as a depression resulting from the anterior growth of the forebrain, and maxillary and mandibular processes: the pericordial swelling constitutes the lower, or caudal, margin. This ectodermally derived invagination which constitutes the stomatodaeum is separated from the upper, or cranial, end of the endodermally derived foregut by the buccopharyngeal membrane (Figure 3.1).

By the fourth week, the buccopharyngeal membrane disintegrates and ectoderm and endoderm intermingle. A similar process occurs at the lower end of the fetal gut with the disintegration of the posterior part of the cloacal membrane, thus joining the hind gut to the proctodaeum and establishing the anorectal canal.

It is difficult to be precise as to the line of demarcation between ectoderm and endoderm in the fully developed mouth due to the intermingling between these two tissues at a primitive stage. The oral mucosa covering lips, cheeks, gingivae and hard palate are derived from ectoderm, as are the teeth, parotid salivary glands and minor labial salivary glands. With the tongue migrating cranially from the tuberculum impar, the lingual mucosa is endodermal in origin. The junction between ectoderm and endoderm is on the floor of the mouth, lingual to lower gingiva and, accordingly, the submandibular and sublingual salivary glands are probably of endodermal derivation. The pharyngeal mucosa, caudal to the pterygomandibular raphe, is entirely of endodermal origin.

The embryonic source of the soft palate and its minor salivary glands remains unclear as this structure develops at the posterior ends of the ingrowing palatal processes, an area corresponding to the earlier junctional zone between ectoderm and endoderm.

39

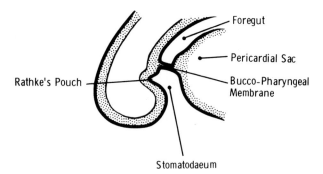

Figure 3.1. Sagittal section of the head and neck region of a three-week-old fetus.

STRUCTURE

The oral mucosa is entirely covered by a stratified squamous epithelium which corresponds to the epidermis of skin. This oral epithelium is separated from the underlying connective tissue lamina propria, equivalent to the dermis, by a basement membrane.

Considerable regional variations exist in the oral mucosa, with respect to whether the epithelium is keratinized or not, the shape of the rete ridges and the structure of the lamina propria.

The oral epithelium can be divided into three broad categories with respect to keratinization: keratinized (lips, gingivae and hard palate); non-keratinized (labial, buccal and alveolar mucosae, soft palate, ventral surface of tongue and floor of the mouth); and gustatory (dorsal surface of tongue), which is a specialized form of keratinized epithelium.

The appendages of the oral mucosae are the minor salivary glands, taste buds and sebaceous glands. The minor salivary glands are numerous on the upper and lower labial mucosae and on the soft palate. Each consists of a few lobules of glandular tissue situated in the submucosal layer with the ducts penetrating the mucosa to open on to the surface (see Chapter 15).

Taste buds consist of ovoid groups of epithelial cells contained within the oral epithelium. In the fetus these buds are widely distributed around the oral mucosa but following birth the numbers decline. In the adult they are most numerous in the lateral walls of the lingual vallate and foliate papillae. Smaller numbers are present on the epiglottis and a few may persist on the soft palate. Impulses transmitting gustatory stimuli are carried in the seventh (VII) cranial nerve for the anterior two-thirds of tongue and in the ninth (IX) cranial nerve for the posterior one-third of tongue and epiglottis.

Ectopic sebaceous glands are commonly found in the oral mucosa although there are no associated hair follicles. These glands appear as small, pale yellowish spots on the lips, and labial and buccal musosae and are of no clinical significance. They have been termed 'Fordyce's spots'.

Sensations of touch and pain from the oral mucosa are carried in the fifth (V) cranial nerve; the maxillary division carrying impulses from the upper half of the mouth and the mandibular division the lower half. The junction between the two divisions runs horizontally along the buccal mucosa.

DISORDERS OF DEVELOPMENT

Developmental disorders vary in their frequency of occurrence. Other than Fordyce's spots and cleft palate, they are generally rare phenomena, although accurate epidemiological data are lacking.

Fordyce's Spots (Fordyce's Granules)

As has been stated above, these ectopic sebaceous glands (Figure 3.2) are of no clinical significance.

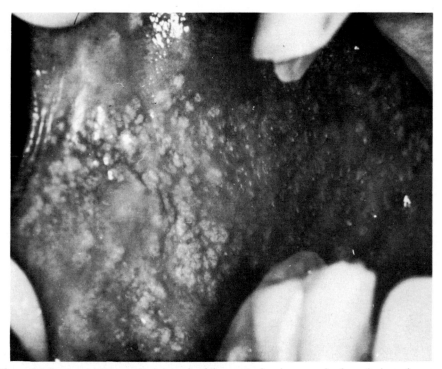

Figure 3.2. Fordyce spots: a marked example of these ectopic sebaceous glands on the buccal mucosa.

Cleft Palate, Hare Lip and Bifid Uvula

These defects are discussed in Chapter 16.

Cleft Tongue (Bifid Tongue)

Embryologically, the tongue is formed by the mid-line fusion of two lateral tubercles. Should this be incomplete the tongue may either be bifid or else have a very pronounced median cleft. This disorder may occur in isolation or in combination with a cleft palate.

Clinical. A deep median cleft or bifid tongue may give rise to problems in eating and speech. Food and debris may accumulate in the cleft and cause irritation.

Histology. In the depth of a cleft, the papillae tend to be absent. Plasma cells and lymphocytes, as evidence of chronic inflammation, may infiltrate the lamina propria.

Treatment. This depends on the severity and symptoms but the fault is readily amenable to surgical correction.

Median Rhomboid Glossitis

This is probably a disorder of development due to the persistence of the tuberculum impar which should be submerged beneath the lateral aspects during the development of the tongue. However, as the lesion often first appears in adulthood, it may represent a local area of chronic inflammation caused by infection with Candida or other micro-organisms. It is more common in males than in females.

Clinical. Median rhomboid glossitis is symptomless and appears clinically as a raised, ovoid- or rhomboid-shaped, smooth red area in the mid-line, anterior to the circumvallate papillae (Figure 3.3). A squamous carcinoma may, rarely, resemble this lesion clinically and a biopsy should be taken if the diagnosis is in any doubt.

Histology. The affected epithelium is devoid of filiform papillae and is hyperplastic with marked downgrowth of the rete ridges. The underlying lamina propria is often infiltrated by lymphocytes and plasma cells and is usually excessively vascular.

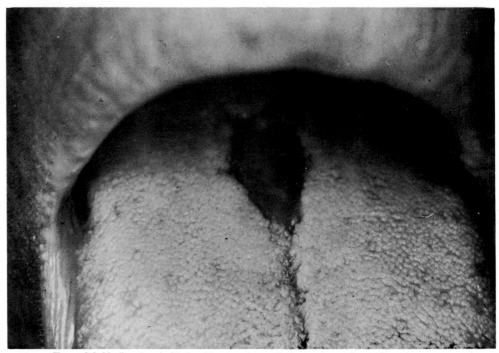

Figure 3.3. Median rhomboid glossitis, showing typical smooth area in mid-line of tongue.

Treatment. As the lesion is symptomless and of no clinical significance, only reassurance is required. However, superficial infection, if present, should be treated by appropriate chemotherapy.

Fissured Tongue (Scrotal Tongue)

Normally, the tongue has some fissures, notably the median fissure, on the dorsum. The degree of fissuring may be accentuated and the condition is then described as fissured tongue (Figure 3.4). The fissuring tends to become more pronounced after puberty and may have a genetic basis. It is also a feature of the Melkersson—Rosenthal syndrome (see below).

Clinical. Prominent fissures which run transversely, sagittally and obliquely are present on the dorsum. No symptoms are associated with this condition.

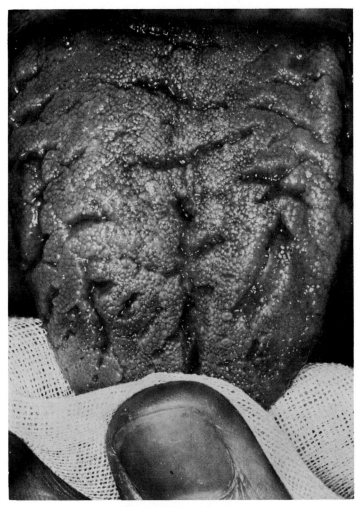

Figure 3.4. Fissured tongue.

Histology. Deep fissures involving normal gustatory epithelium are present.

Treatment. Reassurance, together with advice on maintaining good hygiene in the deeper fissures, is all that is required.

White Sponge Naevus

This relatively uncommon disorder is usually first noticed after birth or in early infancy: it does not develop in adulthood. In most cases it is considered to have a genetic basis with the mode of inheritance being autosomal dominant but exhibiting incomplete penetration. For further consideration of this disorder see Chapter 10.

Sublingual Varices

Dilated veins or varices are commonly seen on the ventral surface of tongue and become increasingly prominent with age. They are of no clinical significance and any patient who comments about these should be reassured.

Focal Epithelial Hyperplasia (Heck's Disease)

This is a condition of unknown aetiology, though both genetic factors and viral infection have been proposed. Children are affected more commonly than adults.

Clinical. Focal epithelial hyperplasia is symptomless and presents as multiple, small (1 to 5 mm diameter) papules on the oral mucosa. These may become nodular and then their colour is similar to that of the adjacent oral mucosa.

Histology. The papular areas appear as discrete lesions exhibiting acanthosis and epithelial hyperplasia. The surface may exhibit hyperkeratosis and parakeratosis. An infiltration of lymphocytes is often present between the elongated rete ridges.

Treatment. The condition is symptomless and the patient may be quite unaware of the presence of these small papules. The lesions regress spontaneously and no treatment is indicated.

Peutz—Jegher's Syndrome (Intestinal Polyposis)

The lesions of Peutz—Jegher's syndrome are present from birth and the disorder is inherited in an autosomal dominant mode but with incomplete penetration. In addition to intestinal polyposis, oral and perioral pigmentation occurs (see Chapter 11).

Epidermolysis Bullosa

This is an uncommon disorder in which the skin and mucosae develop bullae. Several forms of epidermolysis bullosa are recognized, varying both in mode of inheritance and in severity. These are, in order of increasing severity:

1. Epidermolysis bullosa simplex (autosomal dominant)
2. Dystrophic epidermolysis bullosa (autosomal dominant)
3. Dystrophic epidermolysis bullosa (autosomal recessive)
4. Epidermolysis bullosa letalis (autosomal recessive)

For further consideration of this disorder see Chapter 10.

Benign Familial Chronic Pemphigus (Hailey—Hailey Disease)

This uncommon condition may be considered as a disorder of development in that it is transmitted genetically. For further details see Chapter 10.

Melkersson—Rosenthal Syndrome

The triad of features in this rare, apparently genetically determined, condition is facial paralysis, swelling of the lips and a fissured tongue.

Clinical. The disease usually appears in childhood, being intermittent initially but often progressing to an irreversible state. Facial nerve paralysis (Bell's palsy) involves one or both sides and is possibly the result of pressure upon the facial nerve as it emerges from the stylomastoid foramen. The dorsum of the tongue is fissured and rough in only half of those affected and this feature is not essential for diagnosis. The lips become swollen but do not pit on applying pressure. The swelling is painless and may appear in other parts of the mouth as well as in the respiratory tract or on the skin. There is a distinct similarity to the oral manifestations of Crohn's disease but in the latter the neurological signs are absent (see Chapter 11).

Histology. Microscopic examination of the swollen lips or mucosa reveals a sarcoid-like granulomatous reaction and perivascular infiltration of lymphocytes and plasma cells.

Treatment. There is no specific treatment for the neurological disorder. Repeated intralesional injections of depot forms of corticosteroids (e.g. triamcinolone acetonide, triamcinolone hexacetonide, methylprednisolone acetate) tend to reduce the granulomatous reaction in the mucosa. Such injections may be painful and the prior injection of lignocaine into the site is advisable. Due to the relative non-specific nature of the granulomatous inflammation, it is prudent to examine the patient for evidence of sarcoidosis and Crohn's disease.

Fibromatosis Gingivae (Hereditary Gingival Fibromatosis)

Generalized fibromatosis of the gingivae may arise either as an inherited disorder by way of an autosomal dominant gene or as a consequence of drug therapy, notably with diphenylhydantoin (Epanutin, Dilantin) which is used in the treatment of epilepsy.

Clinical. The gingival fibromatosis of the inherited disorder is of fairly rapid onset, usually occurring in combination with the eruption of the secondary dentition. The proliferation of the gingivae may be of such magnitude as to engulf the crowns of the erupted teeth completely. This hyperplastic tissue is obviously subject to trauma as well as inflammation in the pseudo-pockets and therefore is often erythematous in comparison to the normal gingiva.

Histology. The essential morphological feature is fibrous hyperplasia, with numerous coarse bundles of collagen. Epithelial hyperplasia and acanthosis may be evident in the overlying stratified squamous epithelium.

Treatment. The effect of surgical excision tends to be disappointing as the fibromatosis recurs. Careful oral hygiene is necessary in order to minimize the predisposition to gingivitis.

The only definitive treatment of gingival fibromatosis where the mass of tissue is unacceptable is to extract the teeth. This procedure is usually followed by a return to a normal state.

Albright's Syndrome

The triad of features in this syndrome is fibrous dysplasia, endocrine disorder and pigmentation of the skin and oral mucosa. It is not inherited and appears equally in both sexes.

Clinical. Patchy, brown areas of pigmentation on the oral mucosa have been described in this disorder although these are rarer than the cutaneous café-au-lait patches. Endocrine disturbances appear early in life and affect the pituitary, thyroid, para-thyroid and ovaries: precocious puberty in females is a common finding. Polyostotic fibrous dysplasia involves the bones of the face as well as the limbs. (For further details of clinical appearance and treatment, see Chapter 16.)

Non-Odontogenic Cysts

A cyst is defined as an abnormal cavity, containing fluid or semi-fluid material, which is usually lined by epithelium. The non-odontogenic cysts develop from epithelial remnants often left along lines of fusion of the processes which form the face in embryonic development. These cysts are:

Nasopalatine (incisive canal) cyst, medial alveolar and median palatal cysts
Median mandibular cyst
Globulomaxillary cyst (no longer recognized as a fissural cyst)
Nasolabial (naso-alveolar) cyst
Epidermoid and dermoid cysts
Thyroglossal duct cyst
Branchial cleft (benign cervical lymphoepithelial) cyst

The nasopalatine, median mandibular and globulomaxillary cysts, being cysts within bone, are considered in Chapter 16.

Nasolabial (Naso-alveolar Cyst)

This is a rare soft-tissue cyst which occurs in the nasolabial fold and which is thought to arise at the junction between the lateral nasal process and the globular and maxillary processes. Nasolabial cysts are more frequent in females than in males. They appear after puberty and most commonly in middle age.

Clinical. A soft swelling appears in the nasolabial fold, occasionally forming a bulge into both the nostril and the upper sulcus. Radiographs may reveal surface resorption of the underlying alveolar bone.

Histology. The cyst lining may consist of pseudostratified columnar ciliated epithelium, stratified squamous epithelium or cuboidal epithelium.

Treatment. The treatment for nasolabial cysts is surgical excision using an intra-oral approach.

Epidermoid and Dermoid Cysts

These cysts are believed to arise from ectoderm which is enclaved at the time of fusion of the branchial processes. Dermoid cysts are often found in the floor of the mouth and develop during adulthood.

Clinical. Dermoid cysts present as soft swellings under the tongue in the floor of the mouth. Median dermoid cysts, situated above the geniohyoid muscle, produce most swelling on the floor of the mouth and may interfere with eating and speaking due to elevation of the tongue. The lateral dermoid cysts, situated laterally to the genioglossus and geniohyoid muscles, cause a less prominent intra-oral swelling in the region of the sublingual gland: they may also bulge downwards into the submental region. Some dermoid cysts develop entirely below the myelohyoid muscle and present as a swelling in the neck.

These cysts are painless, unless they become infected, and are described as dough-like or fluctuant upon palpation.

Histology. The histology of this group of cysts is variable. If the cyst is lined by a keratinized stratified squamous epithelium containing no other appendages (namely, sebaceous glands, hairs or sweat glands) within its wall it is described as epidermoid. In contrast, a dermoid cyst has skin appendages in its wall. Finally, a complex teratoma may exist, containing stratified squamous epithelium and appendages, bone, muscle and even teeth; that is, structures arising from all three germ layers.

Treatment. The treatment of dermoid cysts is surgical excision.

Thyroglossal Duct Cyst

This is a cyst which may develop from remnants of epithelium at any point along the thyroglossal duct or tract, between the foramen caecum on the dorsum of the tongue and the suprasternal notch. Thyroglossal duct cysts occur at all ages, but are most common in adolescents and young adults.

Clinical. Symptoms depend upon the site of the cyst, which will be either in the mid-line or adjacent to it. When the cyst develops in the tongue it can give rise to dysphagia and bouts of choking. Like most cysts, the thyroglossal duct cyst is painless unless infected. However, fistula formation is not uncommon and about half of the patients experience recurrent infections. A useful diagnostic feature is that this cyst is usually elevated upon protruding the tongue or swallowing.

Histology. The wall of the cyst may be lined with stratified squamous epithelium or pseudostratified columnar ciliated epithelium. Occasionally, the fibrous connective tissue cyst wall contains foci of thyroid tissue.

Treatment. The treatment of a thyroglossal duct cyst is careful surgical dissection and excision.

Branchial Cleft (Benign Cervical Lymphoepithelial) Cyst

The branchial cleft cyst most probably originates from epithelium entrapped in cervical lymph nodes, as does the benign tumour, adenolymphoma, and not from remnants of the branchial arches (hence the preference for the term 'benign cervical lympho-epithelial cyst'). However, doubt remains as to the precise origin.

Clinical. The cyst presents as a painless, slow-growing swelling in the neck. Only rarely, when it bulges upwards from the submandibular region, does it produce an intra-oral swelling.

Histology. The cyst is lined mainly with stratified squamous epithelium which may be replaced in areas by a pseudostratified columnar epithelium. The cyst wall consists, for the most part, of lymphoid tissue together with a small amount of fibrous connective tissue.

Treatment. Careful surgical dissection is necessary as the lesion may recur from any remnants left behind.

MISCELLANEOUS LESIONS

Recurrent Oral Ulceration

Some varieties of oral ulceration are characterized by a tendency to recurrence at the same or at different sites in the mouth. It is convenient to consider these as a group, and the varieties of ulceration which are characterized by recurrence are listed here:

1. Minor aphthous ulceration
2. Major oral ulceration
3. Herpetiform ulceration
4. Oral ulceration in Behçet's syndrome

For more detailed information on each, see below in this chapter.

Other varieties of ulceration may also recur, although, in some cases, this feature is less characteristic of them, or their appearance or associations allow their separation from the list given above. These other varieties are:

1. Traumatic ulceration (see section later in this chapter). This form of ulceration may recur if the cause of the trauma is not identified and removed.

2. Chemical ulceration (see section later in this chapter). Ulceration due to the application of chemicals may recur if its true nature is not recognized and advice to cease application of the harmful chemical has therefore not been given.
3. Erosion associated with disorders of skin and mucous membrane, such as lichen planus and pemphigus (see Chapter 10). These lesions are referred to as erosions rather than ulcers because of their shallowness. They are listed here because the patient with these diseases may complain of recurring ulcerations and fail to mention preceding bulla or association with other change(s) in the mouth. However, they can be differentiated from true ulceration by clinical examination and by appropriate investigation.
4. Ulceration associated with gastrointestinal disease such as ulcerative colitis and Crohn's disease (see Chapter 11).
5. Iron and vitamin B_{12} deficiencies (see Chapter 6).

Minor Aphthous Ulceration (Aphthous Stomatitis, Recurrent Aphthae)

This is a common disease which affects women about twice as frequently as men, and which affects children as well as adults. The aetiology is unknown although simple trauma may excite an ulcer in an ulcer-prone patient. In some patients, the ulcers appear rhythmically and are related to the menstrual cycle, tending to appear in the luteal phase of the cycle. Stressful situations in life cause exacerbation of the ulceration but possible causes, such as bacterial and viral infection and simple allergy to some foodstuff, which have been suggested as aetiological in the past, have not been substantiated by investigation. It is important that those patients whose ulceration is associated with vitamin B_{12}, folic acid or iron deficiency should be recognized and provided with suitable treatment *after* appropriate investigation to elucidate the cause of the deficiency. Minor aphthous ulceration often occurs in more than one member of a family, suggesting a genetic basis as a possibility in aetiology.

Regardless of the basic aetiology, there is a substantial basis for the belief that the ulcers are produced by means of an immunological response. Patients with the disease have a raised titre of circulating antibody, chiefly IgM in type, to fetal oral mucosa. They also possess, in their peripheral blood, lymphocytes sensitized to fetal oral mucosa, suggesting the implication of a type IV hypersensitivity mechanism in causing the disease. Thus evidence exists to support the suggestion that an immunological response to the patient's own mucosa (an autoimmune response) or a cross-reaction between microbial and mucosal antigens is responsible for the localized tissue destruction and ulceration.

Clinical. Recurrent aphthae characteristically appear on the non-keratinized surfaces of the mouth (i.e. buccal and labial mucosa, ventral surface of tongue, floor of mouth and soft palate) as well as on the dorsum of the tongue (Figure 3.5). They are exceedingly rare on the attached gingiva or hard palate and ulcers in these regions should be diagnosed only with caution as aphthae. Aphthous ulcers usually do not exceed 5 mm in size and are round or oval in shape. Healing occurs in less than two weeks without scarring. They are painful, the discomfort often preceding the ulceration.

Histology. The earliest changes occur in the corium where there is mononuclear cell accumulation around small blood vessels. Lymphocytes appear and the mononuclear cells invade the basal layers of the epithelium. Later, large numbers of polymorphonuclears are present and, after localized destruction of the epithelium, an ulcer is formed, the base of which is covered by a fibrinous exudate. At this stage the ulcer has a relatively non-specific appearance.

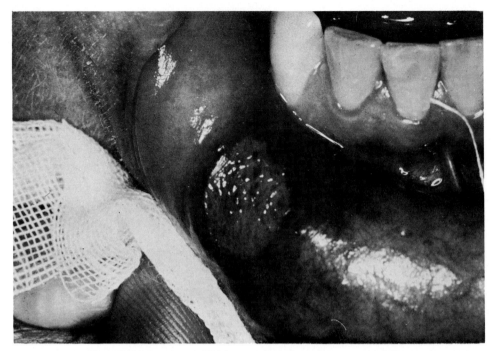

Figure 3.5. Large ulcer on labial mucosa in patient with recurrent aphthae.

Major Aphthous Ulceration (Major Oral Ulceration, Periadenitis Mucosa Necrotica Recurrens).

It is generally believed that major aphthous ulceration represents a severe form of minor aphthous ulceration with an aetiology similar to that described above. Both forms may coexist in one individual at one or at different times. Major aphthous ulcers are larger than the minor ulcers: they may be 10 mm or more in diameter and persist for 4 to 10 weeks. They occur on keratinized and on non-keratinized surfaces and heal with scarring. Patients with recurrent oral ulceration should be asked about possible gastro-intestinal or other disease symptoms. Haematological tests for folate, B_{12} and iron status should be routine (see Chapter 6).

Herpetiform Ulceration

This form of ulceration is quite distinct from intra-oral herpetic infection which is described in Chapter 4. Herpetiform ulceration resembles acute herpetic infection in that up to 100 ulcers may be present at one time during the bouts of ulceration. These occur on keratinized and non-keratinized surfaces and may coalesce to form large ulcers which heal with scarring. Electron microscopic studies have suggested the possibility of a viral infection as the basis of this disease but the aetiology of the disorder is not understood at present.

Treatment. Possible sources of trauma, such as sharp cusps and ill-fitting intra-oral appliances, should be eradicated as far as possible. Topical antiseptics may be used as a mouthwash, particularly in the herpetiform variety, not with the intention of preventing the development of ulcers but to minimize secondary microbial infection of the ulcerated area and thus to relieve the discomfort and facilitate healing. For this purpose, a 0.2 to 0.5 per cent aqueous solution of chlorhexidine gluconate is effective as a mouthwash when used two to four times daily. In the past, antibiotics have been used topically, instead of antiseptics, for this purpose but these may promote candidal infection and their use is to be discouraged.

Mild astringent mouthwashes, such as zinc sulphate (B.P.C.), relieve the discomfort in some individuals and may be helpful if an antiseptic is ineffective.

Corticosteroids are effective in some instances. Two preparations which do not appear to cause adrenocortical suppression are 2.5-mg pellets of hydrocortisone (Corlan) and triamcinalone acetonide in a paste (Adcortyl in Orabase) which adheres to the mucosa for up to 10 minutes. Both of these may be used up to four times daily, the latter as thin or sparing applications. Higher doses of corticosteroids must be used with caution and for limited periods only. A mouthwash made by mixing soluble beta-methasone tablets (Betnesol) with 15 ml of water may be used occasionally. When corticosteroids are advised, due notice must be taken of the dose employed, the period of administration of the drugs and contra-indications to their use.

Oral Ulceration in Behçet's Syndrome

Behçet's syndrome affects the mouth and the skin, genital mucosa, eyes, heart, blood vessels, respiratory system, joints and nervous system in some cases. It affects males more often than females and cannot be recognized on the basis of the oral ulceration which may mimic any of the three forms of recurrent oral ulceration described above. The disease is a hazard to health and life, causing blindness, other serious sequelae and, sometimes, even death.

Treatment. Patients with Behçet's syndrome are best cared for by a general physician and ophthalmologist, although local treatment for recurrent aphthae may be helpful in some cases. However, systemic corticosteroids are the main form of therapy.

Ulceration Due to Trauma

Trauma provided by ill-fitting intra-oral appliances, or biting, is a common cause of intra-oral ulceration. Usually the cause is obvious and the treatment is simple in nature. Occasionally, trauma occurs, unknown to the patient, after use of a local anaesthetic in dental treatment. Recurrent lip or cheek biting may produce a more chronic ulcer or keratosis and the diagnosis may be less obvious. Such chronic irritation may be a cause of localized fibrous hyperplasia. Difficulty is sometimes experienced in differentiating a chronic traumatic ulcer from a neoplastic ulcer. The site and shape of the traumatic ulcer relate precisely to the source of the trauma and the ulcer should heal in one to two weeks when the trauma is removed. However, biopsy is mandatory if there is any doubt in the clinician's mind as to the diagnosis.

Ulceration Due to Burning

Not infrequently the mouth is burnt when very hot food is eaten. The patient may appear with a blister or ulcer in the palate, or elsewhere if the palate is protected by a denture. The diagnosis is obvious after simple questioning. Some patients (known as 'asbestos mouths' to their friends) always consume food which is too hot and may develop localized or generalized forms of stomatitis or ulceration as a consequence. Simple advice, if accepted by the patient, results in cure.

Ulceration Due to the Application of Chemicals

A wide variety of chemicals used by patients in self-treatment of oral complaints, or applied in dental practice or taken accidentally, may cause oral ulceration. Tablets such as aspirin, when held against the oral mucosa, may cause ulceration or formation of a thick white plaque of semi-necrotic keratin and epithelium. Patients with ulceration or any form of stomatitis should always be questioned carefully about the remedies they have employed and about other recent use of chemicals within the mouth, and consideration should be given to the possibility that their disorder is due to these.

Treatment. Application of the offending chemical should be discontinued and replaced by a bland mouthwash. The patient should be reviewed after one week since confirmation of the diagnosis is by healing when the cause is removed.

Geographic Tongue (Benign Migratory Glossitis)

This is a disorder of unknown aetiology which affects both sexes and all age groups. It has been postulated that there may be a psychosomatic background in some cases although a familial tendency has also been demonstrated in others.

Clinical. Benign migratory glossitis presents clinically on the dorsum of the tongue as reddened, smooth areas (Figure 3.6) which are surrounded by a prominent cream-coloured margin. The lesions start as roundish areas, about 1 cm in diameter, but these enlarge and may coalesce, obtaining an irregular outline. The pattern of involvement varies with time. On close inspection of the red patches, small knobbly projections, which are the fungiform papillae, are visible in the red areas. The affected tongue is often fissured.
  The condition may be symptomless but some patients complain of discomfort, particularly when taking hot or spicy foods. If a patient with geographic tongue develops tenderness, other causes of glossitis should be considered, since geographic tongue and nutritional deficiencies may coexist.

Histology. In the central area there is atrophy of the epithelium with the disappearance of the filiform papillae. However, the fungiform papillae remain. At an early stage the epithelium is infiltrated by polymorphonuclear cells which accumulate in small spaces in the superficial epithelial layers.

Treatment. The condition is benign and remains resistant to treatment. Some patients who complain of tenderness respond to an astringent mouthwash, such as zinc sulphate.

Hairy Tongue

Hypertrophy of the filiform papillae leads to the appearance of hairiness on the dorsum of the tongue. The aetiology of this condition is unknown: many factors have been incriminated but no convincing evidence has been established.
  It is more common in males than females.

Clinical. The dorsum of the tongue, particularly the central region, is covered in a mat of fine, hairy projections. These may be white, yellowish or even dark brown. The variation in colour is probably due to staining from diet and smoking as well as from chromogenic bacteria. It is not a painful condition but patients may complain of gagging and of the unpleasant appearance.

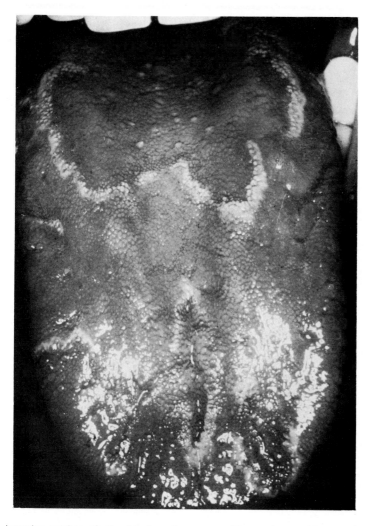

Figure 3.6. Irregular patches of atrophic lingual mucosa with prominent white margins as seen in geographic tongue.

Histology. There is marked elongation of the filiform papillae with numerous micro-organisms entrapped between them.

Treatment. No specific therapy exists for a hairy tongue. The dorsum of the tongue should be kept clean by gentle brushing with a toothbrush. In cases where the papillae grow to an extreme length some individuals have resorted to clipping but the patient must be discouraged from any action which may injure the tongue. The patient should be advised as to the innocent nature of this disorder and encouraged to accept it.

FURTHER READING

Dolby, A. E. (1975) Chapter 9 in Dolby, A. E. (Ed.) *Oral Mucosa in Health and Disease*. Oxford: Blackwell.
Hamilton, W. J. (1975) Chapter 2 in Cohen, B. & Kramer, I. R. H. (Eds.) *Scientific Foundations of Dentistry*. London: Heinemann.
Lever, W. F. & Schaumberg-Lever, G. (1975) *Histopathology of the Skin*. London: Lippincott.
Squier, C. A., Johnson, N. W. & Hackemann, M. (1975) Chapter 1 in Dolby, A. E. (Ed.) *Oral Mucosa in Health and Disease*. Oxford: Blackwell.

chapter 4

_____

Infections

Viral Infections
Bacterial Infections
Fungal Infections

VIRAL INFECTIONS

Herpes Simplex (Type 1)

Virtually all adults have antibodies to this DNA virus, indicating that they have had a primary infection at some point in their lives. There may be a clear history of primary herpetic stomatitis but in most cases it is probable that some oral discomfort during infancy, together with a mild constitutional upset, was erroneously ascribed to the physiological process of teething!

Clinical. Oral infections due to herpes simplex may be divided into primary and secondary conditions. The initial infection with herpes simplex (primary herpetic stomatitis) varies in severity but can be associated with widespread intra-oral vesicles and ulceration (Figure 4.1). It commonly occurs in infancy or childhood, although this may be delayed into early adulthood. With the widespread oral vesiculation and ulceration, the child finds eating painful and loses his appetite. The cervical lymph nodes become enlarged and tender. The child is febrile, fractious and sleeps poorly for the 10 to 14 days over which the condition lasts. On rare occasions, in babies or in children with infantile eczema, the disease is a hazard to life and the virus may also cause encephalitis.

In individuals who have already experienced primary herpetic stomatitis, albeit of a very mild nature, herpes simplex usually presents as an uncomfortable, vesicular lesion on or around the lips (secondary herpes, herpes labialis, cold sore) (Figure 4.1). Various precipitating factors may be involved, including exposure to sunlight, trauma, episode of influenza, fever, psychological stress or menstruation. Presumably all of these factors act either by changing the general immune status temporarily or else by altering the epithelium of the lip. Secondary herpes may also, uncommonly, occur intra-orally as a localized area of vesiculation followed by ulceration. Such lesions represent a difficult diagnostic problem.

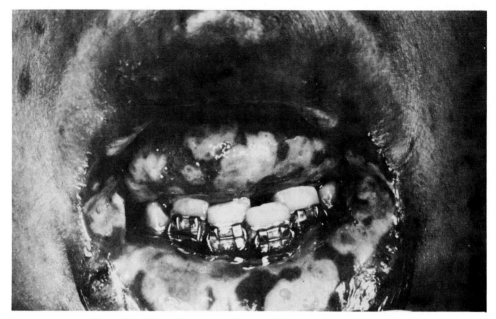

Figure 4.1. Primary herpes simplex stomatitis. Extensive oral ulceration.

Current evidence suggests that the herpes simplex virus, following initial infection, is established permanently and most probably resides in the trigeminal ganglion whence it migrates down the sensory nerves to the lip. This would account for the constancy of site on any one particular lip if just one group of nerve fibres were involved.

Patients who have an incompetent immune response as a consequence of leukaemia, immunosuppressive or cytotoxic therapy tend to develop oral and perioral herpetic infections. In such cases, the herpetic lesions may spread extensively and be most difficult to manage.

The diagnosis of herpes simplex infections is often based on the clinical features but can be established rapidly by the isolation and growth of the virus in cell cultures. In addition, cytological examination of the contents of a vesicle may reveal ballooning degeneration of epithelial cells with intranuclear viral inclusions (Lipschütz bodies) and abnormally large and misshapen nuclei.

A rising serum antibody titre to herpes simplex can be demonstrated: blood is removed during the acute phase of the infection and then about two weeks later in the convalescent phase. An elevation of at least fourfold is considered to be diagnostic.

Treatment. For primary herpetic stomatitis the treatment is empirical. The diet should be soft foods or even just liquid: it is important to encourage fluid-taking as the patient, being febrile, requires fluid replacement. Analgesics, such as paracetamol (U.S. acetaminophen) elixir, are useful and if the child is not sleeping a sedative should also be prescribed: promethazine elixir or dichloralphenazone syrup are suitable. The doses must be related to the child's age.

The oral ulceration is liable to secondary bacterial infection and this may be treated with an antiseptic mouthwash, four to six times daily. A mouthwash of 0.2 to 0.5 per cent aqueous chlorhexidine has the advantage of being an effective antiseptic as well as inhibiting plaque accumulation upon the teeth. As such, the gingival condition will be maintained when toothbrushing is difficult and painful. An alternative mouthwash is

0.5 to 1 per cent povidone-iodine (Betadine). This is another effective antiseptic but is not effective in inhibiting plaque formation.

Idoxuridine dissolved in dimethylsulphoxide is an antiviral agent which acts topically. Cytosine arabinoside has also been used for this purpose. Antiviral agents are not usually required in herpetic stomatitis or in herpes labialis, but these agents may be of use where there is extensive cutaneous spread, or in immunodeficient patients. Here the concentrations of idoxuridine used can vary from 5 to 40 per cent, depending upon the response.

Herpes labialis responds reasonably to the repeated topical applications of ether, 70 per cent ethanol, or 0.5 per cent chlorhexidine in 70 per cent ethanol. Topical steroids should not be used for the treatment of herpes simplex as there is the potential danger of depressing the local immune reaction and hence of encouraging a spread of the infection.

Herpes Zoster

The herpes zoster virus is responsible for chickenpox in children and shingles in adults (Figure 4.2).

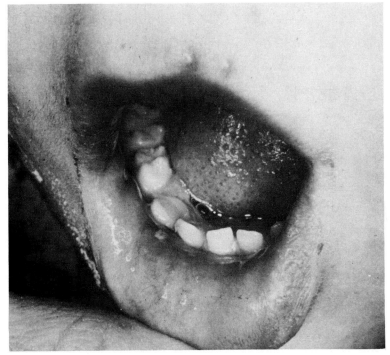

Figure 4.2. Chickenpox (herpes zoster infection). Typical skin vesicles and some ruptured oral vesicles are shown.

Clinical. Chickenpox is characterized by cutaneous vesicles and these may also appear on the oral mucosa. This is of little clinical consequence.

Shingles presents as a unilateral lesion, confined to the distribution of a nerve. The trigeminal nerve involvement causes intra-oral lesions which may be localized to the distribution of the maxillary or mandibular divisions. Vesicles appear on one side of the oral mucosa and these soon rupture leaving tender ulcers. Pain is a characteristic feature of shingles, usually preceding the eruption, and is sometimes sufficiently severe to require narcotic analgesics.

The vesicles and ulcers clear within two to four weeks but, particularly in older people, post-herpetic neuralgia can be most persistent and distressing, continuing in some cases for as long as two years (see Chapter 21).

Treatment. The oral manifestations of chickenpox usually do not cause any symptoms and, accordingly, no treatment is required. Should the ulcers be painful then a 0.2 per cent aqueous chlorhexidine or 1 per cent povidone-iodine mouthwash can be used four times daily.

Shingles is best treated as soon as possible by painting the vesicles with idoxuridine, 5 to 40 per cent, in dimethylsulphoxide six times daily. In the mouth, a gauze swab can be moistened with the preparation and held in contact with the mucosa. The drug amantadine (Symmetrel) is considered to act by preventing certain viruses from penetrating cells. It is useful in the treatment of shingles and reduces the incidence of post-herpetic neuralgia. The dose is 100 mg twice daily for two to four weeks.

Coxsackie

These RNA viruses are associated with two disorders of the mouth, namely herpangina and hand, foot and mouth disease.

Clinical. Herpangina is a condition caused by infection with coxsackie A virus. It is usually confined to children and presents as widespread small ulcers on the mucosa together with a fever and general malaise. The oral symptoms may be preceded by a sore throat or conjunctivitis and the disease is self-limiting in 10 to 14 days. As such, the disorder is very similar to primary herpetic stomatitis, but the two conditions can be differentiated either by isolation of the virus or by a rising antibody titre. It is probable that herpangina is another one of the febrile states of childhood where the aetiology is commonly attributed to 'teething'.

Hand, foot and mouth disease is caused specifically by coxsackie A-16 virus and is also usually confined to children. Along with a constitutional upset, including mild fever and nasal congestion, a papular or vesicular rash appears on the upper and lower limbs. Vesicles appear on the oral mucosa and these soon ulcerate, leaving painful lesions. The distribution of the oral lesions in hand, foot and mouth disease differs from primary herpetic stomatitis in that the gingivae are not often involved. The disease is self-limiting within 14 days.

Treatment. There is no specific treatment for oral coxsackie infections. Treatment should be empirical, as for primary herpetic stomatitis, and an antiseptic mouthwash, soft or liquid diet, analgesics and sedatives should be used as necessary.

Measles

The incubation period for measles is 8 to 10 days, and the onset of the disease is marked by the eruption of a maculo-papular rash on the skin. A few days prior to the appearance of the cutaneous lesions the patient becomes febrile and shows symptoms of respiratory infection and conjunctivitis. In this prodromal phase, small whitish granules or spots with an erythematous margin (Koplik's spots) may be seen on the buccal mucosa. These are of no clinical significance other than for diagnostic value and no treatment is required.

Infectious Mononucleosis (Glandular Fever)

It seems likely that infectious mononucleosis is caused by the Epstein—Barr virus. This is a disorder of children and young adults and may present as a trivial fever or as a more serious and prolonged illness with lymphadenopathy, fever, headaches, general malaise and hepatosplenomegaly. Infectious mononucleosis is diagnosed by the Paul—Bunnell heterophile agglutinin test, an elevated lymphocyte count and the presence of atypical lymphocytes in the blood.

Clinical. The oral manifestations of infectious mononucleosis may resemble those of acute primary herpetic or coxsackie stomatitis with widespread mucosal ulceration. In addition, petechial haemorrhages and ecchymoses may be present, particularly on the palate.

Treatment. There is no specific treatment for the oral manifestations of infectious mononucleosis. A soft diet and antiseptic mouthwash (aqueous chlorhexidine) should be used while the oral lesions last. The use of ampicillin should be avoided in these patients as it frequently leads to a rash.

Reiter's Syndrome

This is a disorder of young adults, predominantly males, for which the aetiology remains unknown, although the disorder is thought to be due to an infective agent. The lesions of Reiter's syndrome are urethritis, arthritis, conjunctivitis and oral ulcers or erosions (see pages 206-207).

Clinical. Oral manifestations develop in a variable number of cases and take the form of red, granular patches, which may have a whitish margin, on the mucosa.

Treatment. As the aetiology is uncertain, there is no specific treatment for Reiter's syndrome and the management should be undertaken by a general physician. Tetracycline and corticosteroids have been used with some success.

BACTERIAL INFECTIONS

Tuberculosis

There has been a reduction of the incidence of infections due to *Mycobacterium tuberculosis* in most countries. Oral involvement is relatively infrequent and when it does occur it is usually secondary to open pulmonary tuberculosis.

Clinical. Tuberculosis of the oral mucosa presents as a persistent ulcer which gradually increases in dimension. The outline tends to be irregular and the ulceration may be superficial or deep. The tongue is most commonly involved but lesions may appear on any part of the oral mucosa.

On general examination there is likely to be evidence of pulmonary infection and the patient may give a history of malaise, weight loss, haemoptysis and intermittent fever. However, the oral lesions may occur as part of a primary infection or in miliary tuberculosis.

Any ulcer suspected of being tuberculous should be biopsied, as indeed should any ulcer of more than four weeks' duration. Histology would reveal a granulomatous reaction with chronic inflammatory cells, giant cells and epithelioid cells. Necrotic foci may also be present. Special stains, particularly using immunofluorescent techniques, may reveal mycobacteria in the lesion. Microbiological investigation of swabs from the ulcer and of sputum should be undertaken in order to identify the organism, together with appropriate radiological and other investigations to determine the extent of the infection. A general medical examination, including chest x-ray, should be arranged.

Treatment. The treatment of the oral lesions of tuberculosis is that of the underlying infection with appropriate chemotherapy and antibiotics.

Scarlet Fever

Scarlet fever is a disorder of children which is caused by a toxin produced by beta-haemolytic streptococci which are present as an upper respiratory tract infection.

Clinical. A widespread erythematous appearance develops in the oral mucosa and this is accompanied by an erythematous, cutaneous rash, fever and headaches. The tongue undergoes a series of characteristic changes: initially the dorsum develops a whitish coating through which red, oedematous fungiform papillae project. This is described as a 'strawberry tongue'. Subsequently, the white coating is shed and the dorsum becomes smooth and erythematous but for the enlarged fungiform papillae. This stage is termed a 'raspberry tongue'. By two weeks from the commencement of symptoms the oral manifestations and rash have generally cleared.

Treatment. There is no specific treatment for the oral manifestations of scarlet fever. Management is directed towards the condition in general.

Infection of Angular Cheilitis

Angular cheilitis may be due to a nutritional deficiency (see Chapter 6) or, more commonly, to an inadequate vertical dimension caused by missing teeth or defective dentures. The latter leads to constant wetting of the fissures at the angles of the mouth, the skin of which eventually becomes macerated and cracked. Secondary infection commonly occurs, aggravating and perpetuating the condition (Figure 4.4e).

The organisms commonly involved are *Staphylococcus aureus* and *Candida albicans* and, less often, beta-haemolytic streptococci. Any of these organisms may exist alone or in combination with the others.

Treatment. The management of angular cheilitis should be directed towards identifying the basic aetiological factor. However, swabs and smears should be taken from the fissures and any pathogenic organisms identified together with their sensitivity to antibiotics. Staphylococcal infections usually respond to the topical application of tetracycline or fucidic acid (Fucidin) ointment six times daily. Topical use of neomycin on the skin may cause an allergic dermatitis and should not be used. Candidal infections are treated with an appropriate antifungal drug, e.g. amphotericin B or nystatin.

As it is impossible to differentiate clinically between the infections of staphylococci and candida and because the infection in angular cheilitis is frequently mixed, it may be necessary to use an antibiotic and an antifungal agent combined. Surprisingly few preparations are available. Some contain neomycin or else are combined with a corticosteroid and are probably unsuitable. Two per cent miconazole cream (Daktarin) is indicated, as this single agent is effective both against candida and gram-positive cocci.

In cases where candidal infections are present, it is wise to administer antifungal lozenges concurrently in order to eradicate the potential reservoir of these micro-organisms in the mouth.

With regular application of an ointment and eradication of infection, many cases of angular cheilitis will improve, albeit temporarily, until the aetiological defect is controlled.

Syphilis

Syphilis may affect the mouth in the primary, secondary or tertiary phases of the disease.

Clinical. The primary chancre develops at the site of inoculation and most frequently occurs in the genital organs. In a number of cases, however, the mouth is affected and the chancre may be found on the lips or tip of tongue, although any other mucosal site may be involved.

On the lips, the chancre appears as a firm nodule with an ulcerated top which may be crusted. Intra-orally, the chancre is similar but the ulcerated area is covered by a greyish slough. *Treponema pallidum* can be readily obtained from the chancre surface and, accordingly, the chancre is highly contagious. Characteristically, cervical lymphadenitis is present. The chancre heals in one to two months.

At about two to four months after the primary stage, a cutaneous rash develops and ulceration of the oral mucosa may occur as the secondary stage of the disease. This involvement of the mouth takes place regardless of the site of primary infection. The oral ulcers are superficial, with a greyish slough, and have been described as 'mucous patches'. These are also highly infectious and *Treponema pallidum* can be isolated from the patches and seen under the microscope with dark field illumination, although it must be remembered that other spirochaetes can be found within the mouth. Serological tests for syphilis are positive by this stage.

The intra-oral ulcers clear up within a few weeks although recurrences may occur intermittently over a few years.

Tertiary syphilis develops after several years have elapsed and is marked by gummata and luetic glossitis. A gumma is a granulomatous reaction with central necrosis and appears in the palate or tongue. Gummata may reach several centimetres in size and these ulcerate leaving a necrotic base. This process may eventually lead to palatal perforation.

Chronic glossitis with interstitial fibrosis may also develop in the tertiary stage and these cases are thought to have a greater incidence of leukoplakia and squamous carcinoma (Figure 4.3).

Gonorrhoea

Gonococcal infection of the mouth arises as a consequence of orogenital contact where gonococcal urethritis or cervicitis already exists in the partner. Such a history is rarely forthcoming and the diagnosis is difficult.

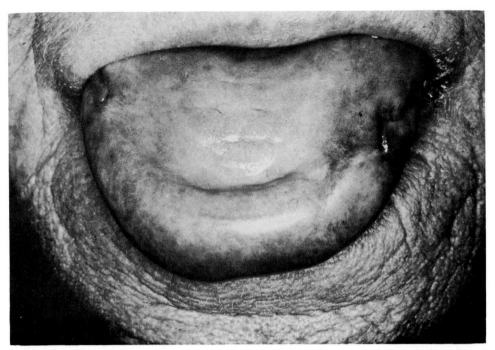

Figure 4.3. Tertiary syphilis. Papillary atrophy and interstitial fibrosis of tongue. There is ulceration of the lateral margins.

Clinical. Gonorrhoea of the mouth may present as a non-specific stomatitis or pharyngitis and it is probable that many cases are misdiagnosed. Where there are persistent superficial ulcers on the mucosa it is worth taking a swab and examining it for the characteristic intracellular gram-negative diplococci.

Treatment. This is similar to the treatment of genital gonorrhoea. Penicillin, tetracyclines and co-trimoxazole are all used and therapy should last for five days.

Actinomycosis

The anaerobic *Actinomyces* is responsible for abscesses in the region of the mouth and neck and does not cause a disorder of the mucosa as such.

The diagnosis is made upon the appearance of colonies of the organisms, which resemble sulphur granules, in the pus and in the culture of the *Actinomyces*.

Actinomycosis is treated by prolonged treatment with antibiotics, usually penicillin.

FUNGAL INFECTIONS

Candida albicans

Candida albicans is found in more than 50 per cent of the mouths of healthy adults in the absence of any evidence of infection. Certain factors, local and systemic, permit this commensal micro-organism to cause disease. Local factors such as ill-fitting appliances or inadequate care of an appliance may be at fault. In other cases, systemic factors such as pregnancy, corticosteroid therapy, diabetes mellitus, blood dyscrasia, immune deficiency or suppression, general debility, Addison's disease, iron deficiency and hypoparathyroidism predispose to the infection. Administration of broad spectrum antibiotics may suppress the bacterial flora of the mouth, facilitating overgrowth of *Candida albicans* and candidosis, and the topical use of antibiotic lozenges or a mouthwash may have a similar effect.

Clinical. Candidosis may present in a variety of forms (Figure 4.4). Pseudo-membranous candidosis (thrush) is the accumulation upon the mucosa of soft white plaques which can easily be rubbed off with a blunt instrument, leaving an erythematous and bleeding base. These white plaques of masses of candidal hyphae occur on any part of the oral mucosa. Severe forms of pseudomembranous candidosis may be associated with ulceration and may, with difficulty, be distinguished from other forms of severe acute stomatitis causing marked discomfort.

In atrophic candidosis, the mucosa appears bright red and thin, without either keratotic white patches or a white pseudomembrane upon the surface. This condition is characteristically seen under dentures, especially on the palate, where the term 'denture stomatitis' or 'denture sore mouth' has been applied. In these cases, the micro-organisms proliferate on the fitting surface of the denture and presumably release noxious factors which, directly or indirectly, cause the atrophic and inflammatory reaction in the mucosa. In diagnosis of pseudomembranous candidosis or atrophic candidosis, smears should be taken for direct examination in addition to swabs for microbiology. The smears, which are studied by gram stain, are examined for the filamentous hyphal forms of *Candida*. Less commonly, other forms of *Candida*, e.g. *Candida krusei*, may be responsible and these do not form hyphae. Swabs confirm the presence of *Candida* but, as has already been stated, up to half of the population have this micro-organism in the oral cavity as a normal commensal. In atrophic candidosis, swabs should always be taken from the fitting surface of the upper denture.

Chronic hyperplastic candidosis resembles other white patches in the mouth and cannot be rubbed off. The white patch does not have the reticular appearance of lichen planus but may have a speckled erythematous appearance although this is not a constant feature. The disease may affect the dorsum of tongue or the buccal mucosa, close to the angle of the mouth. Histology reveals hyperparakeratosis and epithelial hyperplasia and variable atypia: acute and chronic inflammatory cells are present within the lamina propria and polymorphs also invade the stratified squamous epithelium. Hyphae of *Candida* can be demonstrated in the cornified layers of the epithelium. The pathogenesis of chronic hyperplastic candidosis is still unclear. It does appear to be somewhat more common in patients with a nutritional deficiency (iron and folate), suggesting that the yeasts invade an already abnormal epithelium. Sometimes there is difficulty in deciding whether candidal infection has caused the lesion or has invaded a pre-existing leukoplakia. In any event it does seem that candidal infection, per se, can produce tissue changes similar to those described as chronic hyperplastic candidosis.

Angula cheilitis has already been discussed. Candida are frequently secondary invaders of the established fissures at the commissures.

Treatment. Where there is any suspicion of an underlying systemic disorder, the appropriate investigations should be initiated. This is particularly important in cases of recurrent candidosis.

Pseudomembranous candidosis is treated by allowing one amphotericin B lozenge or nystatin tablet to dissolve in the mouth four times daily. For children, a suspension of

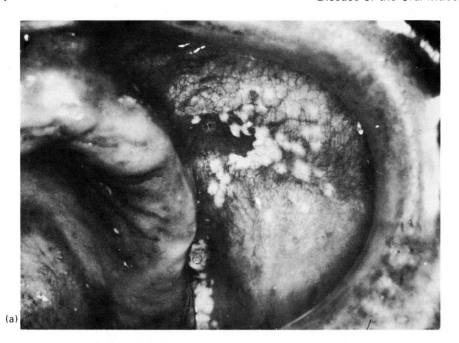

(a)

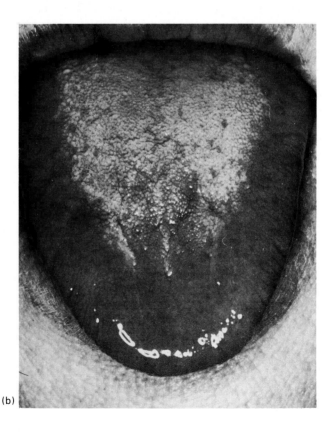

(b)

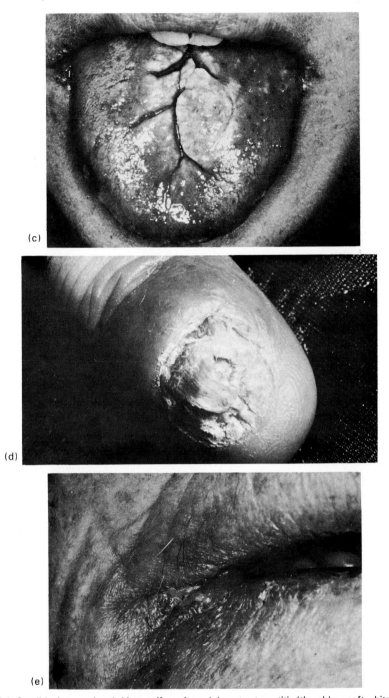

(c)

(d)

(e)

Figure 4.4. Candidosis — oral and skin manifestations: (a) acute stomatitis (thrush) — soft white patches on buccal mucosa induced by steroid drug therapy; (b) acute stomatitis — atrophic inflamed borders of tongue induced by antibiotic drug therapy; (c) chronic hyperplastic — white adherent patches on dorsal surface of tongue; (d) chronic mucocutaneous — infection and inflammation of nail matrix (onychia) and area around nail bed (paronychia); (e) angular cheilitis — infection and grooving of lip angles often associated with denture stomatitis.

amphotericin, nystatin or natamycin is available and there is little to choose between these although nystatin tends to be the least pleasant. Atrophic candidosis is treated in a similar manner, but attention must also be paid to regular cleansing of the dentures. An anti-fungal cream should be smeared on the fitting surfaces of the dentures four times daily. This ensures a high and prolonged local action. Ill-fitting dentures are either corrected or replaced.

When *Candida* is involved in angular cheilitis, an anti-fungal cream should be rubbed into the fissures six times daily. Where there is the possibility of a mixed infection or doubt about the organisms at all, as is often the case in general practice, then miconazole cream is recommended.

The management of chronic hyperplastic candidosis often poses a more difficult problem. Even after months of topical therapy the lesion may not resolve. This could represent either a problem of penetration of the anti-fungal agent into the epithelium or, alternatively, a situation where *Candida* had possibly invaded a pre-existing leukoplakia. The further possibility exists that patients do not persevere with treatment. In these cases, removal of the persistent hyperplastic patch may be advisable.

Histoplasmosis

Infection with histoplasma is characterized by fever, lymphadenopathy and hepato-splenomegaly. A productive cough and arthritis may also exist.

Clinical. The intra-oral manifestations of histoplasmosis are nodules upon the mucosa together with ulcers. The ulcers start by being round or oval but may coalesce to form an irregular area. The margins tend to be slightly raised or rounded.

Treatment. Amphotericin is used systemically for the treatment of histoplasmosis but there is no specific or reliable agent.

Other Fungal Infections

A number of other fungal infections may affect the oral mucosa but they are rare and confined to certain regions. These include blastomycosis, coccidioidomycosis and cryptococcosis.

FURTHER READING

Burnett, G. W. & Scherp, H. W. (1976) *Oral Microbiology and Infectious Disease*. Baltimore: Williams and Wilkins.
Juel-Jensen, B. E. & MacCallum, F. O. (1972) *Herpes Simplex, Varicella and Zoster. Clinical Manifestations and Treatment*. London: Heinemann.
Walker, D. M. (1975) Chapter 11 in Dolby, A. E. (Ed.) *The Oral Mucosa in Health and Disease*. Oxford: Blackwell.

chapter 5

Tumours and Premalignant Lesions

INTRODUCTION

Many different types of neoplasms affect the oral cavity. Benign and malignant neoplasms may arise from oral mucosa, bone, salivary glands and the odontogenic apparatus. In addition, metastasis from distant primary sites may involve the oral cavity.

Recent information from regional cancer registration centres has indicated that approximately 80 to 90 per cent of all oral malignancies are squamous cell carcinomas. The elderly are those predominantly affected and the incidence and mortality rate increase with each decade. It is interesting to note that oral cancer mortality rates vary from country to country. In South East Asia, especially India and Ceylon, oral carcinoma has a high prevalence among the malignant neoplasms. There appear also to be site variations: thus, in France, carcinoma of the buccal mucosa has a relatively high prevalence. Male/female ratios may also vary: for example, in France the ratio is 8:1 in comparison with 3:1 for England and Wales. In many countries, the incidence of oral carcinoma and the mortality rate associated with it appear to be declining gradually. There is also a suggestion that, for some sites, the male preponderance is disappearing.

BENIGN TUMOURS AND TUMOUR-LIKE LESIONS

Squamous Cell Papilloma

The squamous cell papilloma is a benign epithelial neoplasm observed at times in the oral cavity. The mucosae of the cheek, gingivae, palate, lips and tongue are equally affected (Figures 5.1 and 5.2). The lesions vary in colour from pale pink to white and in size from a few millimetres upwards. They have either a sessile or pedunculated attachment to the oral mucosa. As a consequence of trauma during mastication the lesions may become ulcerated and infected. All age groups are affected though the lesions are most commonly seen in the elderly. No epidemiological data are available to indicate the frequency of occurrence of squamous cell papillomas, and there is no evidence to suggest they are premalignant. The occurrence of multiple papillomas in association with verruca vulgaris of the skin is observed from time to time, especially in children with the habit of finger-sucking. Whether papillomas have a viral aetiology is still unknown. Histologically, the squamous cell papilloma presents a characteristic appearance of keratinized stratified squamous epithelium thrown into folds and supported by a vascular connective tissue stroma.

The treatment consists of complete surgical excision.

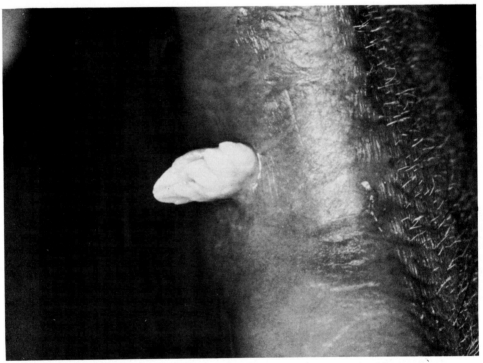

Figure 5.1. A squamous cell papilloma on the oral mucosa at the angle of the mouth.

Keratoacanthoma

This benign lesion occasionally occurs at mucocutaneous junctions and rarely in the mouth. It is primarily a skin lesion which, histopathologically, shows a characteristic crater plugged with keratin and enclosed by hyperplastic epithelium. The keratoacanthoma is considered to originate by hyperplasia of a hair follicle together with squamous metaplasia of the associated sebaceous gland. Keratoacanthoma is a self-limiting lesion which may resemble squamous carcinoma clinically and histologically.

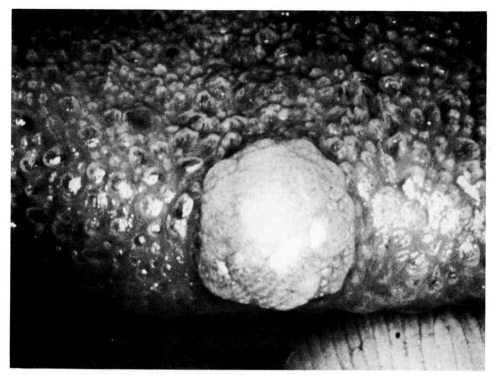

Figure 5.2. A squamous cell papilloma affecting the tip of the tongue.

Pigmented Naevus

Pigmented naevi occur in the oral mucosa, presenting as small brown raised areas in the buccal mucosa, gingiva, lip and palate. Such lesions are not common. It is worth noting that like their counterparts in the skin, the lesions are not always pigmented. There are three types of pigmented naevi: dermal, junctional and compound. The principal cell type of the dermal naevus is the naevus cell which is ovoid in shape, has a hyperchromatic nucleus and contains a variable amount of melanin. These cells are arranged in clusters within the connective tissue of the corium. The junctional naevus comprises proliferating melanocytes forming cell clumps in the region of connective tissue—epidermal interface. In the compound naevus, the melanocytes appear to migrate from the junctional area with the result that cords of cells are present both in the basal epithelial layer and in the corium.

Children and young adults are most commonly affected. Malignant transformation, though it may occur, is extremely rare.

Fibroma and Fibrous Swellings

Fibrous overgrowths of oral soft tissues are common conditions, often related to trauma, and usually occurring in response to chronic irritation. A true fibroma is probably rare, although the clinical separation of this from fibrous overgrowth can be difficult, if not impossible.

Fibrous swelling can occur anywhere in the oral tissues, although the gingiva is the commonest site. Such swellings have a slow rate of growth and are painless unless traumatized. A gingival growth is termed 'fibrous epulis'. The lesion may be sessile or pedunculated and may be quite vascular in an early phase of its development. Long-standing lesions are firm, pale and relatively avascular. Lesions of tongue, lip and buccal mucosa tend to present as small nodules (fibro-epithelial polyp). Palatal and alveolar lesions are often associated with ill-fitting dentures and range in appearance from small fibrous tags to large, irregular exophytic growths (Figure 5.3). Such a swelling is usually described as denture fibroma or denture granuloma.

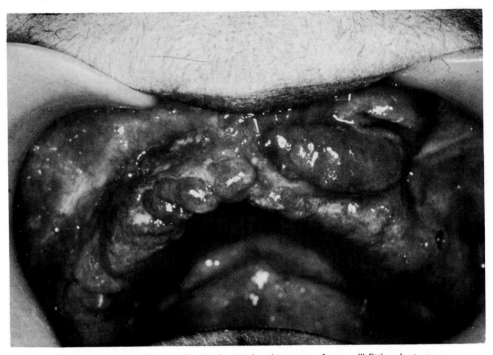

Figure 5.3. Overgrowth of fibrous tissue related to trauma from an ill-fitting denture.

A true fibroma comprises dense collagen bundles with a peripheral condensation of tissue assuming the appearance of a pseudocapsule. The fibrous overgrowth or swelling is less well organized and the collagen bundles are irregularly arrayed without a pseudo-capsule. The early lesion may be highly vascular, composed of vascular granulation tissue infiltrated by polymorphs, mononuclear cells and lymphocytes. Such a swelling is usually described as a pyogenic granuloma. It may gradually fibrose.

The lesions are best treated by removal of the irritant and surgical excision of the lesion.

Certain unusual forms of fibromatosis or more extensive fibrous enlargement of oral structures are described in the paragraphs that follow.

Pseudosarcomatous fasciitis is an uncommon condition which affects hands and abdomen and, rarely, the oral cavity. Histologically, the features suggest fibrosarcoma but the lesion is fundamentally benign and comprises vascular, highly cellular connective tissue.

The nasopharyngeal fibroma is an unusual lesion which affects young males. It manifests as a lobulated mass of tissue arising from the soft tissue of the nasopharynx. Histologically, fibrous connective tissue with a marked vascular element is noted. Nasal obstruction and epistaxis are common presenting symptoms and recurrence after excision is likely.

Gingival fibromatosis is a benign condition characterized by a general, firm swelling of the gingival mucosa. Histologically, fibroblastic proliferation together with mucoid degeneration may be observed. The swelling may be so marked as to cover the child's teeth and a familial incidence has been reported. The fibromatosis may be associated with other developmental defects.

Diffuse gingival enlargement may occur, albeit uncommonly, in leukaemia, and may also be caused by certain anti-epileptic drugs, such as phenytoin (e.g. Dilantin, Epanutin; see Figure 5.4). In contrast, a more common cause is chronic inflammation, as occurs in gingivitis and periodontitis due to local factors such as plaque accumulation.

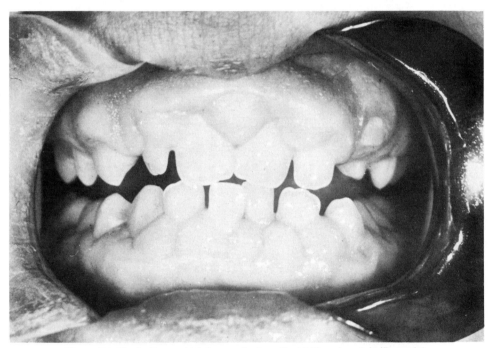

Figure 5.4. Gingival hyperplasia in an epileptic patient taking phenytoin (Epanutin).

Lipoma

The lipoma is a common benign neoplasm but it occurs infrequently in the mouth, usually as a solitary rounded soft swelling beneath buccal mucosa.

Haemangioma and Lymphangioma

Haemangioma is a common vascular swelling which is best considered as a hamartoma rather than a true neoplasm, implying that it results from an error in development. The lesion may be classified according to histological type: cavernous, capillary, or mixed forms. The haemangioma may occur on any part of the skin or oral mucosa (Figure 5.5). The companion lesion, the lymphangioma, particularly affects the tongue and buccal mucosa (Figure 5.6) and small lymph-filled sinusoids project from the surface as transparent swellings.

Multiple angiomatous lesions may contribute to Sturge—Weber syndrome, Rendu—Osler—Weber syndrome and Maffucci's syndrome.

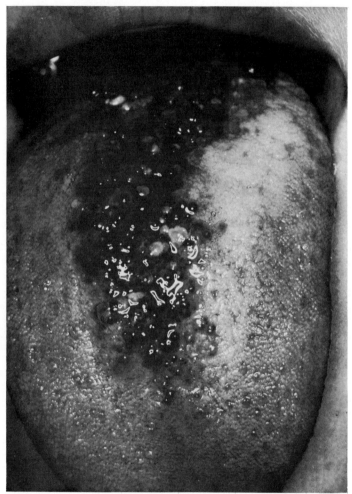

Figure 5.5. Haemangiomatous lesions affecting the dorsal surface of the tongue in an eight-year-old child.

Nerve Tumours

The neurilemmoma is a tumour of the peripheral nerve sheath and may occur as an asymptomatic swelling in any part of the oral cavity. Histologically, slender, elongated, spindle-shaped cells are arranged in a whorled fashion and sometimes show palisading with their nuclei arranged parallel to each other like a row of soldiers. Occasionally, these cells form a reticular microcystic pattern. The tumour is encapsulated.

Neurofibromas are most probably developmental abnormalities rather than neoplasms, and they incorporate all parts of the nerve, including its sheath. The lesion is usually solitary, although multiple forms may be encountered, and on rare occasions plexiform varieties of these may be associated with malignant medullary thyroid tumours. Multiple neurofibromas also occur in neurofibromatosis (von Recklinghausen's disease of nerve) and form obvious subcutaneous and submucosal nodules. Patchy melanistic pigmentation of the skin appears and patients with this disorder should have a blood-pressure check since the disorder may be associated with the adrenal medulla tumour phaeochromocytoma. The nodules in neurofibromatosis may show malignant transformation occasionally.

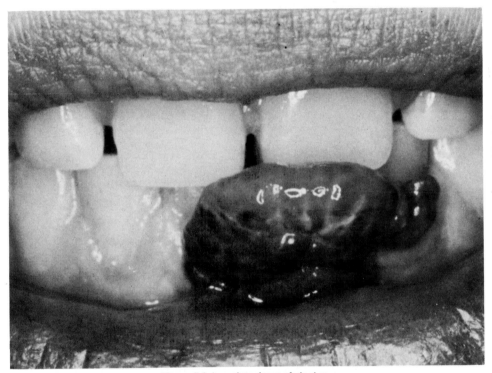

Figure 5.6. Lymphangioma of gingiva.

The traumatic neuroma is not a true neoplasm but an overgrowth of nerve fibres following severance of a nerve. It represents an exaggeration of the normal reparative process and may give rise to pain.

MALIGNANT TUMOURS

Squamous Cell Carcinoma

Squamous cell carcinoma accounts for approximately 90 per cent of all oral malignancies.

Clinical and Histological Appearances

Carcinoma of the mouth occurs more commonly in men than in women and middle-aged and old patients are most frequently affected by it. The clinical appearance is variable (Figures 5.7, 5.8 and 5.9) but all areas of leukoplakia and erythroplakia and all ulcers which fail to heal in two to three weeks should be regarded with suspicion. A biopsy is mandatory if the diagnosis of squamous carcinoma is suspected.

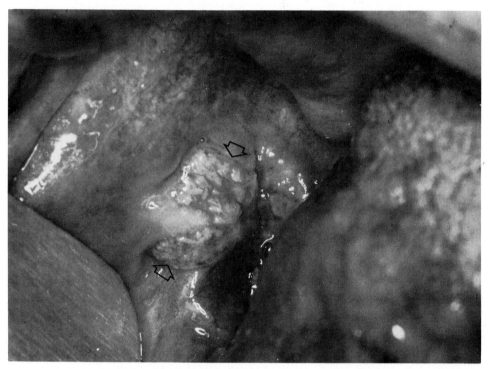

Figure 5.7. Squamous cell carcinoma (arrowed) of buccal mucosa.

The tissues are infiltrated by abnormal epithelium which extends from the surface as sheets or finger-like processes into the underlying corium and muscle. The abnormal cells are usually easily identified as epithelial in nature and show a maturation process comparable to that seen in normal surface epithelium, even to the formation of keratin. Such tumours are described as well differentiated but even in these the cells lack orderly arrangement and show nuclear pleomorphism, hyperchromatism, irregular stratification, and an increased mitotic rate. In poorly differentiated tumours the abnormal tissue is less easily recognized as being of epithelial origin because of a complete lack of order in the arrangement of the cells and a wide variation in size and shape of the cells and their nuclei. The connective tissue stroma of the tumour and surrounding the tumour is usually infiltrated by lymphocytes, suggesting a host response to the invading neoplasm.

Carcinoma of the lower lip is approximately 20 times more common than that of the upper lip. It usually appears as an ulcer although an exophytic form may occur. Such

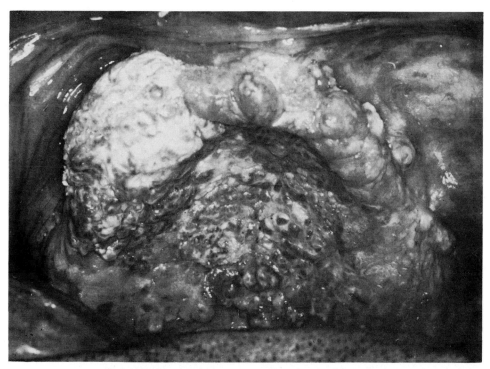

Figure 5.8. An extensive squamous cell carcinoma of the palate.

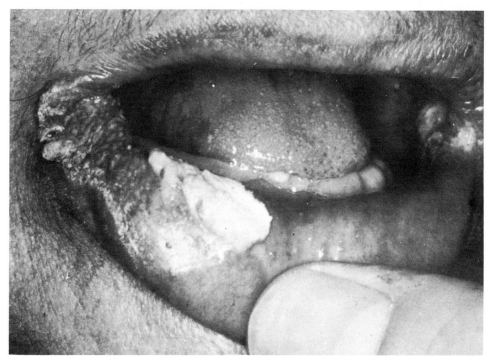

Figure 5.9. A squamous cell carcinoma of the lip.

carcinomas grow and invade rapidly and regional lymph node involvement can occur. Due to the likelihood of early detection, however, the prognosis is generally good with a 90 per cent five-year survival rate. It should be noted that early carcinomas of the lip appear as a scabbed, superficially eroded and slightly indurated area which may resemble herpes labialis with delayed healing.

Carcinoma of the tongue accounts for about 50 per cent of intra-oral carcinomas and may arise in pre-existing leucoplakia. The lateral border of the middle third of the tongue and the ventral surface are the usual sites. The tumour is usually well differentiated histologically but lymph node metastasis occurs early. Less than one half of patients with this disease survive five years after diagnosis.

Carcinoma of the buccal mucosa tends to occur opposite the third molar tooth and it may extend into musculature of the cheek and on to the palate. If detected early the prognosis is good. Only about 10 per cent of intra-oral carcinomas occur in this site.

Carcinoma of gingiva tends to appear in the premolar or molar region and may spread to involve bone, causing loosening of the teeth. It accounts for about 10 per cent of intra-oral carcinoma.

Carcinoma of the floor of the mouth tends to occur anteriorly, beneath the tongue, and appears as an ulcer or wart-like growth. About 15 per cent of intra-oral carcinomas occur on the floor of the mouth.

Carcinoma of the palate usually involves the soft palate. The prognosis at this site is considered to be poor, with a survival rate of less than 5 per cent, but the tumour accounts for only about 10 per cent of intra-oral carcinomas.

Aetiology of Squamous Cell Carcinoma

Many factors have been implicated as causing oral cancer but in most cases no single factor can be identified as the major agent. It seems likely that the disease is caused by many agents and that some of these may act as promotors or cocarcinogens.

Evidence relates pipe- and cigar-smoking to oral cancer. The evidence is less convincing in the case of cigarette-smoking, although it does suggest the possibility of a link. Carcinoma of the mouth and pharynx, as for the lungs, appears more often among smokers than among non-smokers and this is particularly the case with carcinoma of the lip, floor of the mouth and tongue. In some countries, a link between carcinoma of the floor of the mouth and cheroot-smoking in women has been suggested and in parts of India reverse cigarette-smoking is said to be a factor in causing carcinoma of the palate. Tobacco-chewing is recognized as a possible cause of leukoplakia and cancer; and, in some parts of the world, tobacco blended with lime and rolled in a betel leaf is used to form a quid which may be held in the mouth for most of the day. There is an increased risk of oral cancer in persons adopting such habits.

Alcohol may be a contributing factor in causing oral cancer but this seems to be related to the type and quality of beverage rather than its quantity. Crude, home-distilled spirits appear to be especially harmful.

Systemic factors such as iron and vitamin deficiency are difficult to evaluate. They may cause epithelial atrophy. Carcinoma of the upper part of the oesophagus appears to be more likely in iron-deficient patients and this relationship may exist for the mouth, pharynx and other parts of the oesophagus as well.

Syphilis is frequently linked as a causative factor in older reports. It is not clear whether the disease itself was at fault or the various arsenic preparations used in its treatment. Syphilis appears to be less important as a possible aetiological agent nowadays.

Dental decay, chronic infection related to the teeth, and chronic trauma caused by broken teeth and ill-fitting and old appliances are often linked with oral cancer. It is said that the disease rarely occurs in well-cared-for mouths although relatively little clinical experience will provide exceptions to this rule. Some patients with oral cancer have no obvious dental cause; nevertheless, it remains possible that chronic irritation can act as a promoting factor.

Sunlight is probably a factor in causing lip cancers, an idea supported by the knowledge that this tumour affects the lower rather than the upper lip and most frequently affects people involved in outdoor occupations.

Much interest has been directed recently at the possible link between oncogenic viruses and oral cancer. No firm evidence at present links such infection with carcinoma of the mouth, although the possibility requires further study.

The Early Detection of Oral Cancer

As with all diagnosis, the importance of detailed clinical examination, together with a good history, cannot be overstressed. Unfortunately, cancer of the oral cavity is often first diagnosed at a late stage in the development of the disease and, since it has been shown that the size of the tumour at the time of diagnosis influences the prognosis, early diagnosis is to be encouraged.

The early squamous carcinoma may appear as a white patch, erythematous area, fissure, nodule or ulcer. The ulcerated form tends to have a rolled and everted border with an indurated base.

The major clinical signs which mark more advanced oral carcinomas are induration, ulceration and fixation to underlying structures. Elevation of the lesion, together with fungation and mobility of teeth, are additional features. Pain is a late feature of oral cancer, unless infection supervenes or perineural lymphatics are invaded.

Late or advanced oral cancer is characterized by extensive spread to important local structures, giving rise to symptoms such as tongue immobility, trismus, pathological fracture and disturbance of sensory or motor function. Metastatic spread to the regional lymph nodes, often bilaterally, depends upon the tumour site and lymph drainage from the affected area. Ulceration of the primary tumour will of course give rise to infection and reactive hyperplasia of regional lymph nodes.

Verrucous Carcinoma

This distinctive lesion occurs as an exophytic wart-like lesion which grows slowly and invades adjacent soft tissues and bone relatively late in its growth (Figure 5.10). It appears chiefly in patients who are more than 60 years old and is associated with tobacco-chewing and snuff-taking habits. Histologically, the tumour is formed by folded hyperplastic epithelium remarkable for the rounded and much enlarged rete ridges which do not extend deeply into the corium. There is little cellular atypia. The connective tissue is usually heavily infiltrated by a predominantly lymphocytic cell population.

Radiotherapy should be avoided since this may induce frank carcinomatous change. With careful surgical excision the prognosis is good.

Melanocarcinoma

This malignant tumour may arise from a pre-existing junctional naevus or de novo. Although it is uncommon in the mouth, it usually presents there on the maxillary alveolar ridge or palate, both in men and in women, in middle or old age. The tumour appears as a deeply pigmented patch which soon ulcerates and may bleed. Amelanotic forms are also encountered. The tumour is highly cellular, the cells either containing melanin pigment or being free of pigment. The outlook is poor: recurrence, spread to regional lymph nodes, and blood spread to distant sites are to be expected.

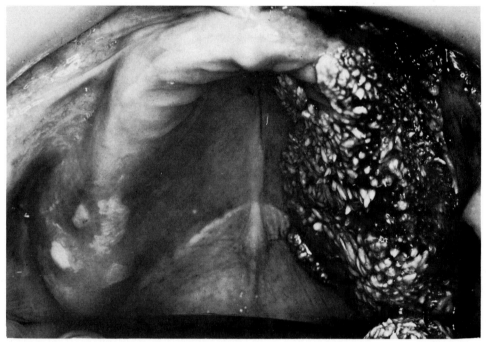

Figure 5.10. A verrucous-like lesion affecting the mucosa of alveolus, and tuberosity. Histologically, the lesion showed features of verrucous carcinoma, although early invasion was noted.

Sarcoma

A sarcoma is a malignant tumour arising from a connective tissue element: fibrous tissue, adipose tissue, muscle, bone, cartilage, and vascular and neural elements may give rise to malignant tumours of this type. The clinical feature is usually a swelling which increases in size over a period of weeks or months, and histology will allow identification of the precise tumour type.

Treatment and Prognosis of Oral Malignant Disease

The choice of available treatments includes surgery, radiotherapy and chemotherapy, either alone or in various combinations. The method likely to be adopted varies from centre to centre and there is, as yet, no particular method which produces a uniformly good result, supported by evidence as to the elimination of the neoplasm, patient survival and quality of life. Most studies give an indication of five or ten years' survival rate and, in interpreting these, the age range of patients must be taken into account.

Clearly, initial site is important with regard to prognosis. Thus, an 80 to 90 per cent, 5-year survival rate can be predicted for carcinoma of the lip compared with 25 to 40 per cent for intra-oral carcinomas. In general, the prognosis is poorer for posterior than for anterior lesions, for tumours which are large or have already spread to the regional lymph nodes when first diagnosed, and for poorly differentiated tumours lacking a good lymphocytic response.

It is now common to 'stage' a tumour clinically when the diagnosis is first made, in order to help assess the various treatment methods and long-term follow up. One system commonly employed is the TNM system: T refers to the primary tumour, N to the lymph nodes and M to distant metastases. TNM categories are available for tumours for different parts of the body. For example, a tumour of the mouth might be categorized as T2, N1, M0, implying that the primary tumour is greater than 2 cm and less than 4 cm in size, there are clinically palpable, homolateral, non-fixed cervical lymph nodes which are suspected to contain metastatic tumour, and there are no distant metastases found on clinical examination.

PREMALIGNANT ORAL LESIONS

Introduction

In some cases, though by no means all, squamous carcinomas are preceded by certain mucosal changes. These changes are often referred to as premalignant because malignant change occurs in them more frequently than can be explained by chance. It must be emphasized, however, that the term 'premalignant' when used in this way does not imply the certainty of malignant change in a definite time-scale: many patients with these mucosal features never suffer any further ill effect.

Lesions which may be premalignant are:

1. Leukoplakia
2. Erythroplakia
3. Lichen planus (see Chapter 10 for details)
4. Oral epithelial atrophy
5. Submucous fibrosis

Leukoplakia

'Leukoplakia' is a clinical term used to describe a slightly raised white patch of 5 mm or more in diameter which cannot be rubbed off and which cannot be diagnosed as any other specific entity on clinical or histological grounds (Figure 5.11).

Some confusion exists as to which conditions should be included under the heading 'leukoplakia' and which should be excluded. For the purposes of this book, some changes with recognized aetiology are described under this heading, but many leukoplakias have no obvious aetiology.

Leukoplakia can be induced by the following:

1. Cigarette-, pipe- or cigar-smoking. Patients who smoke many cigarettes each day often show a generalized slight keratotic change with white plaques on the anterior part of the buccal mucosa, tongue and palate. Patients who constantly dangle a lit cigarette from the lips develop a localized keratosis there. Pipe-smokers may have a localized keratosis on one part of the dorsum of the tongue or palate

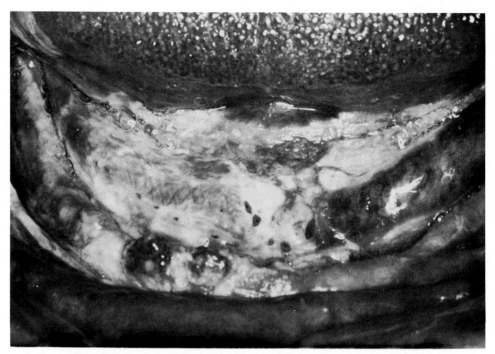

Figure 5.11. Extensive leukoplakia of the floor of the mouth and alveolar mucosa.

related to their favoured pipe position. The thickening of the cornified layer on the palate often causes some obstruction to the ducts of minor salivary glands whose pouting orifices project through the whitened surface as red spots, giving an appearance known as stomatitis nicotina (Figures 5.12 and 5.13).

2. Tobacco-, betel-nut- and other chewing habits. The leukoplakia produced by these chewing habits is often localized to the site favoured by the patient as a holding-place for the tobacco quid or material being chewed. The leukoplakia may be severe and show a tendency to malignant change.

3. Iron, vitamin and other deficiency. The oral mucosa tends to become atrophied in deficiency states and leukoplakia may be added to this change.

4. Syphilitic glossitis. The chronic glossitis which occurs in the tertiary phase of syphilis predisposes to leukoplakia. In the past this was an important premalignant condition which often predated squamous carcinoma. The disease is now uncommon.

5. Candidal leukoplakia (Figure 5.14). Some leukoplakias show superficial infiltration with *Candida albicans*. This may or may not produce a speckled appearance clinically. It is not clear whether the leukoplakia is due to chronic candidal infection or whether this occurs as a complication of the leukoplakia. It is possible that either situation may occur.

6. Frictional keratosis (Figure 5.15). Chronic frictional irritation may cause a white patch which may, or may not, disappear when the cause of the irritation is removed.

7. Alcohol. It is doubtful if alcohol is a significant single factor in causing leukoplakia.

8. Idiopathic. Some leukoplakias have no apparent cause even after exhaustive investigation. Such lesions require most careful treatment since they would appear to show a greater tendency to malignant change than would other leukoplakias.

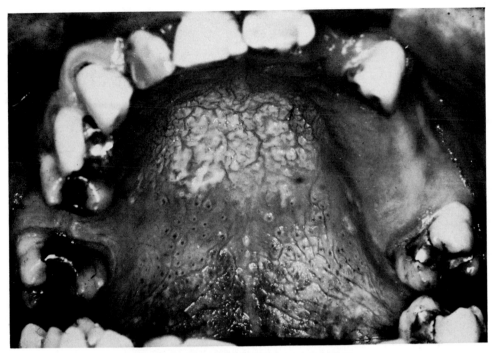

Figure 5.12. Stomatitis nicotina due to pipe-smoking.

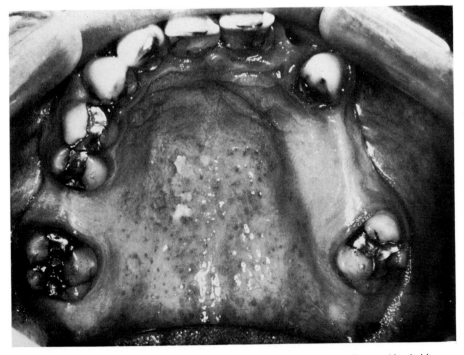

Figure 5.13. Disappearance of stomatitis nicotina after cessation of the pipe-smoking habit.

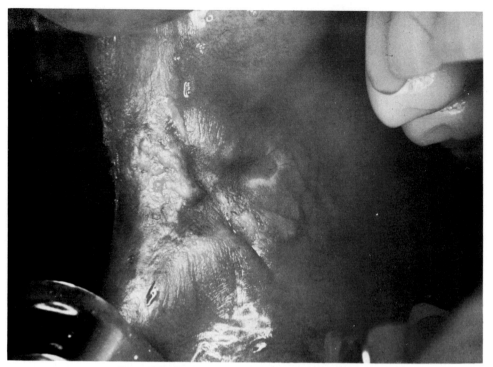

Figure 5.14. Candidal leukoplakia at the angle of the mouth.

Leukoplakia affects men more frequently than women and chiefly patients in middle or old age. The leukoplakia may appear as a thin or thick white patch of varying size on almost any part of the mouth. Some thin patches are almost transparent in quality: other patches remind one of a thick layer of paint. The leukoplakia may have a white speckled form on an erythematous base and such speckled leukoplakias require most careful assessment since they would appear to have a more unfavourable prognosis than other forms. In summary, on clinical grounds, leukoplakia can be described as (a) homogeneous, (b) verrucous (warty), or (c) speckled. Leukoplakia can be felt as a rough or slightly thickened area but it is neither indurated (firm and rubbery) nor fixed to deeper structures. 'Acute leukoplakia', that is a leukoplakia with a short history and showing a tendency to increase in size over a period of weeks, requires immediate biopsy since such a lesion is most likely to be a squamous carcinoma.

The histological features of leukoplakia are a conspicuous surface layer of keratin, a thickening of the prickle cell layer of the epithelium, producing deepening and widening of the rete ridges (acanthosis), and an infiltration of the corium by a variable number of lymphocytes and plasma cells. In candidal leukoplakia and when cellular atypia is marked, flattened, deeply-staining nuclei persist in the keratinized layer; a feature described as parakeratosis in contrast to the more usual orthokeratosis.

It is most important to examine the epithelium for cellular atypia. This term is used when two or more of the following features are present: nuclear hyperchromatism, increased nuclear/cytoplasmic ratio, cellular and nuclear pleomorphism, increased and atypical mitoses which may be sited more superficially in the epithelium than is usual, individual cell keratinization deep in the epithelium, focal disturbance in cell arrangement and adhesion, and basal cell hyperplasia causing drop-shaped rete ridges.

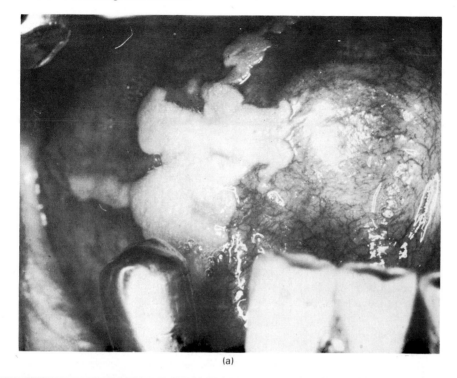

(a)

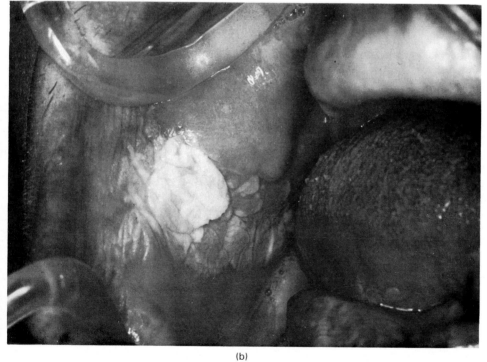

(b)

Figure 5.15. Frictional keratosis: (a) the under-surface of the tongue; (b) the buccal mucosa.

In the past the term 'dyskeratosis' was employed to describe cellular atypia but dyskeratosis may have a variety of meanings and its use is best discontinued. When cellular atypia is marked so that there is abnormality of the full thickness of the epithelium, with no differentiation of cells from basal to superficial layers, a top to bottom change, the condition is referred to as carcinoma in situ. It should be emphasized that leukoplakia, being a clinical term, is not favoured by histopathologists. The histological diagnosis is of keratosis with mild, moderate or severe cellular atypia.

Erythroplakia (Erythroplasia)

This term is used to describe a well-demarcated velvety red patch on the oral mucosa. Inflammation may cause erythema but the term 'erythroplakia' describes a circumscribed lesion which is persistent and usually associated with cellular atypia. The aetiology may be similar to that of leukoplakia and the two conditions may coexist. Histologically, erythroplakic patches have either no surface keratinized layer or a thin surface layer, and usually show marked cellular atypia or the features of carcinoma in situ. They require most careful assessment and management, since they represent the most severe of the oral precancerous lesions, and excision is almost always the treatment of choice.

Oral Epithelial Atrophy

Oral epithelial atrophy is observed in a number of conditions such as syphilis, oral submucous fibrosis, and iron and vitamin deficiencies. Although carcinoma has been reported in association with these conditions, the role of local and systemic factors has not been fully clarified. Treatment of epithelial atrophy is treatment of the underlying cause.

Submucous Fibrosis

Oral submucous fibrosis is a disease which is almost entirely confined to adults of Indian origin. The aetiology is unknown but the disease may be associated with use of chillis, a potent spice commonly used in India. The patient complains of a burning sensation and vesicles or ulcerations may be apparent on intra-oral examination. Later, submucous fibrosis occurs. The lips are immobile and the patient cannot open the mouth for more than a few centimetres. The mucosa at this stage is pale and the constraining fibrous bands are obvious on examination.

Histology reveals hyalinization and acellularity of dense fibrous tissue in the corium. Blood vessels are narrowed or disappear and lymphocytes are present in small numbers as an infiltrate. The epithelium is atrophied and cellular atypia may be apparent.

It would appear that patients with submucous fibrosis are more likely to develop leukoplakia and squamous carcinoma than other persons. A further hazard of the condition is that simple dental disease and infection can hardly be treated in a patient who is unable to open the mouth. Thus a dento-alveolar abscess may become a major problem in a person with the disease.

Advice to avoid possible irritants, together with passive opening exercises, perhaps assisted by a spatula or some other simple device placed between the teeth, may be helpful. Local and systemic corticosteroids have been employed by some with at least temporary benefit and surgical measures may be adopted if dense fibrous bands fail to yield to other measures.

The Management of Premalignant Lesions in the Mouth

Proper management of leukoplakia and of other premalignant lesions is based on the identification of likely aetiological factors, the careful recording (diagrammatic and photographic) of clinical appearances and a knowledge of the histology of the lesion. Thus it is necessary to undertake a thorough case history, a careful physical examination of the mouth and, almost always, biopsy of the diseased area. In all cases, aetiological factors which have been identified should be excluded as far as possible. This may entail removing causes of frictional irritation, giving advice regarding smoking and chewing habits, or treating infections such as candidosis or syphilis. The discussion which follows relates to leukoplakia since the treatment of the other premalignant lesions has already been considered.

A choice must be made between active eradication of the leukoplakic area by excision or by cryotherapy and passive observation of the diseased tissue, once the causative factors have been removed as much as possible. Consultation with an oral surgeon is necessary and the decision to remove all that is possible of the leukoplakic area may be encouraged by the following: a small well-demarcated leukoplakia, a readily accessible leukoplakia, leukoplakia of the floor of the mouth (see below), a young or fit patient, focal atypia on histology and carcinoma in situ on histology. In contrast, a more conservative approach and long-term review of the lesion is more applicable in widespread leukoplakia affecting several parts of the mouth, a leukoplakia affecting areas which are 'surgically' difficult, an old or ill patient, absence of cellular atypia on histology, and a good response to removal of causative factors.

In practice, a combination of active intervention and passive observation is applied in many cases, and many leukoplakias are kept under long-term review at regular intervals. Patients are usually seen every three months, although longer intervals are acceptable in some cases. The patient should be encouraged to report 'any change' which takes place between appointments. Many patients imagine that absence of pain denotes a satisfactory state, not realizing that early squamous carcinomas are often painless. It is for this reason that advice is given to report 'any change'. Review appointments provide an opportunity for reiterating advice regarding smoking and other aetiological factors and for making an assessment of the efficacy of the advice already given. The following clinical features, if present at a review appointment, might indicate malignant change and the need for further biopsy: change in the appearance or size of the leukoplakic area, ulceration, fissuring or cracking of the leukoplakia, induration or firmness, erythroplakia, speckling, exophytic growth, clinical or radiographic evidence of bone destruction, if the leukoplakia overlies bone, and enlargement of the regional lymph nodes.

Most patients with leukoplakia will not develop squamous carcinoma and in only about 5 per cent of cases will malignant change occur, in from one to 20 years after the diagnosis of leukoplakia has been made.

Speckled and verrucous leukoplakia, leukoplakia of the tongue and of the floor of the mouth, extensive leukoplakia and cases lacking obvious aetiology would appear to show a greater tendency to malignant change than leukoplakia in general. Leukoplakia showing cellular atypia is especially dangerous but the absence of atypia cannot be regarded as an indication of completely innocent behaviour, particularly in verrucous leukoplakia and in leukoplakia of the floor of the mouth. The behaviour of a leukoplakic patch cannot be predicted with precision and all such patches require careful assessment and management.

FURTHER READING

Cohen, B. & Kramer, I. R. H. (1976) *Scientific Foundations of Dentistry.* London: Heinemann Medical Books.

Dolby, A. E. (Ed.) (1975) *Oral Mucosa in Health and Disease.* Oxford: Blackwell.

Lucas, R. B. (1976) *Pathology of Tumours of the Oral Soft Tissues,* 3rd ed. Edinburgh: Churchill Livingstone.

Shafer, W. G., Hine, M. K. & Levy, B. M. (1974) *A Textbook of Bone Pathology,* 3rd ed. Philadelphia, London, Toronto: W. B. Saunders.

chapter 6

Nutritional Disease

Nutrition — General Comments
Aetiology of Nutritional Deficiencies
General Features of Nutritional Deficiency
General Management of Nutritional Deficiency
Oral Manifestations

NUTRITION — GENERAL COMMENTS

Man requires a diet which not only fulfils the caloric requirements but also includes essential amino acids, fatty acids, vitamins and minerals. The number of calories needed to maintain homeostasis is, in general, proportional to the energy expenditure or physical activity. Depending upon occupation, individuals need from 1500 to 4500 calories per day and this fluctuating demand is most commonly adjusted with a variable intake of carbohydrate.

Although a considerable portion of our diet does consist of carbohydrate, it is in itself not a necessary dietary constituent and is utilized to fulfil the caloric requirement. On the other hand, a diet devoid of carbohydrate, wherein the caloric requirements are met by proteins and fatty acids alone, is not necessarily an optimal diet since, over a prolonged period, it may promote generalized diseases.

A balanced diet is one in which all essential nutrients are ingested within certain limits. The precise quantities will fluctuate from individual to individual as well as under different conditions. In addition to this, if any one nutrient is taken in a quantity outside the specified range it is not unreasonable to expect that the balance of the remaining essential nutrients must undergo a compensatory adjustment. The overall dietary pattern thus regulates the absolute requirements for each specific nutrient.

In general, each society adopts a type of adequate balanced diet dependent upon local resources as well as affluence. Accordingly, it is conceivable that there will be permutations of what constitutes a balanced diet for any one group and this will vary from one part of the world to another. Therefore, although absolute nutritional requirements are published from time to time, these figures should be taken only as approximate guidelines.

Further, there is not usually a simple, precise cut-off point, above which there will be optimal health and below which there will be rampant clinical manifestations. Nutritional deficiencies present to a variable degree and thus have a broad spectrum of severity of symptoms and signs, with the preponderance of clinical manifestations often correlating to the extent of the deficiency.

An additional point which may cause some confusion is that the nutritional deficiency may exist in isolation, such as occurs in the vitamin B_{12} deficiency of pernicious anaemia, or else the patient will present with a group of deficiencies, as in malabsorption or generalized inadequate intake. The precise diagnosis can sometimes be confused by the fact that a primary deficiency of one substance can lead to a secondary deficiency, either due to alteration in the nutritional balance or, alternatively, by changing the absorptive pattern of the intestine: in cases of vitamin B_{12} deficiency there is an apparent decrease in the ability of the intestinal mucosa to absorb folic acid, another vitamin.

AETIOLOGY OF NUTRITIONAL DEFICIENCIES

Deficiencies of essential nutrients may arise in many ways and, as has been stated above, can exist in isolation or in groups. These aetiological factors are classified as follows.

Inadequate Intake

This is simply the situation where the nutritional requirement is not being met by an adequate diet. On a world-wide scale, the commonest reason for this is poverty and lack of education. In the relatively more affluent Western societies it is less common to find individuals who cannot afford an adequate diet. In these communities it is more often the elderly members who, for various reasons, cease to prepare an adequate diet and tend to limit themselves to foods of convenience which frequently consist mainly of carbohydrate in one of its many refined forms. The other section of society in which inadequate intake is a feature is composed of those of low intelligence who have no appreciation of the necessity for a well-balanced nutritious diet and, again, these individuals will often exist on a greater portion of convenient carbohydrates.

Disorders of Digestion

In this group, the actual intake may be reasonable but the nutrients are not assimilated because of a derangement in the digestive apparatus. For food digestion to proceed normally, an obvious requirement is a fully functional alimentary tract. Individuals who have had a gastrectomy or who suffer from achlorhydria, or pancreatic or hepatobiliary disease are prone to deficiency disorders due to inadequate digestion of their dietary intake.

Defective Absorption

With a suitable intake and adequate digestion, the next phase is absorption through the intestinal mucosa. In any disorder in which the bowel wall is affected, such as coeliac disease, regional enterocolitis or ulcerative colitis, or in which the contents pass through the intestine too rapidly, as in chronic alimentary infections with bacteria or amoeba, there is no opportunity to absorb nutrients. This gives rise to a state of malabsorption wherein deficiencies occur in groups.

Alterations in the intestinal bacterial flora by the long-term ingestion of certain antibiotics, e.g. neomycin, can produce nutritional deficiencies because man depends upon a symbiotic relationship with intestinal bacteria which synthesize vitamins.

Finally, under this heading it is convenient to consider the effect of an intestinal parasite utilizing the dietary supply of a nutrient. The prime example of this is vitamin B_{12} deficiency due to infestation by tapeworms.

Alterations in Metabolism

The action of certain drugs, be they antibiotic or cytotoxic, is to influence pathways involved in the further metabolism of specific nutrients. Methotrexate (amethopterin) is a cytotoxic agent used in the treatment of several malignant neoplasms and of leukaemia. The action of this substance is to interfere with folic acid metabolism and patients receiving this form of therapy often develop manifestations of folic acid deficiency.

Increased Metabolic Demands

Changes in the metabolic status of an individual can lead to an increase in the demand for nutrients. During pregnancy there is a substantial increase in the requirements for the developing fetus as well as by the mother herself. The deficiencies most commonly encountered in pregnant women are of iron and folic acid. It is thus a widespread practice to administer supplements of these two nutrients during gestation.

Loss of Nutrient

Loss of nutrients most commonly occurs in the form of an iron deficit due to chronic blood loss. Females, during their decades of menstruation, are perpetually on the brink of becoming iron deficient as a consequence of menstrual bleeding. The degree of blood loss at the menses is variable and although it is relatively simple to diagnose an overt case of menorrhagia it can be somewhat more difficult to decide whether or not the iron deficiency can be ascribed solely to menstruation in a patient who, possibly, has periods which are heavier than normal.

Chronic blood loss from the gastrointestinal tract is relatively common. The insidious, unspectacular trickle from a peptic ulcer or haemorrhoids can be sufficient to produce iron deficiency. Carcinoma of the bowel is another source of intestinal bleeding and must be considered in the absence of other diagnoses.

Renal disease, with long-standing haematuria, is a further possible cause of iron deficiency although this is less common than the other causes of chronic haemorrhage discussed above.

GENERAL FEATURES OF NUTRITIONAL DEFICIENCY

From a consideration of the multiplicity of aetiological factors leading to a nutritional deficiency it is apparent that a patient may appear generally well or, alternatively, present with a series of systemic symptoms and signs which lead one to the correct diagnosis.

Classical descriptions of the clinical manifestations of specific nutritional deficiencies in human beings can sometimes become confused because of the difficulty in establishing precisely which nutrients are missing. Although the status of several nutrients can be measured fairly readily, it is most difficult to obtain an accurate estimate of the tissue content of many others. Hence, in disorders where there is liable to be a group of deficiencies, only those which can be readily measured are recorded.

Other information about the manifestations of deficiencies in human beings has been gathered from administering particular nutrients to patients with deficiencies and observing the effect, particularly noting the improvement of lesions. Finally, animal experiments have been conducted, using synthetic diets which are known to omit only a single nutrient at a time.

GENERAL MANAGEMENT OF NUTRITIONAL DEFICIENCY

When a nutritional deficiency is suspected on clinical grounds, the most obvious step is to confirm this, where possible. The most frequent nutritional deficiencies encountered in Western societies are of iron, folic acid and vitamin B_{12} and the body's status can be estimated by measuring the serum iron and total iron binding capacity, corrected whole blood folate and serum vitamin B_{12}. Other deficiencies are less common and would rarely exist without being reflected in a concomitant lowering of one of the above three nutrients.

Once the presence of a deficiency is established it is certainly inadequate merely to give the patient replacement therapy: an aetiology for the deficiency must be sought in a most vigorous manner. A thorough dietary and medical history should be taken and the patient passed on for a complete medical examination, together with whatever special investigations are indicated. The proper management of a case of nutritional deficiency is to uncover the aetiological factor and correct the basic underlying problem, and only when this has been accomplished can a decision regarding the necessity for replacement therapy be made.

If the patient has any distressing symptoms attributable to the nutritional deficiency, such as oral ulceration or angular cheilitis, it is reasonable to alleviate these with a topical regimen of therapy but one which would not interfere with the studies aimed at elucidating the nature of the basic underlying disorder.

For oral ulceration, it would be reasonable to prescribe a 0.2 per cent aqueous chlorhexidine mouthwash, four times daily, to eradicate secondary infection from the ulcers and so facilitate healing. Angular cheilitis, when due to a nutritional deficiency, would be treated at this initial stage by the application of an appropriate topical antibacterial or antifungal preparation, depending upon the organisms infecting the fissures.

ORAL MANIFESTATIONS

The oral mucosa appears to be very sensitive to disturbances in nutritional status and may often develop the first apparent signs of a deficiency. As such, careful examination of the mouth is of the utmost importance in any case where there is the least suspicion of a deficiency. Similarly, it is important that any intra-oral examination, especially a routine dental check-up, should include the soft tissues. When such an approach is adopted oral lesions, indicative of the more sinister underlying disease, may be detected.

A considerable amount has been written in an attempt to differentiate between various specific deficiencies from the nature of the oral lesions. From the present evidence we are not convinced about the specificity of many intra-oral lesions and believe that further work is required in this field. Glossitis, angular cheilitis and oral ulceration (Figures 6.1—6.3) have been attributed to several different deficiencies and the only practical approach to adopt in these cases is an all-encompassing series of investigations. This, together with a careful medical history and examination will usually clarify the situation.

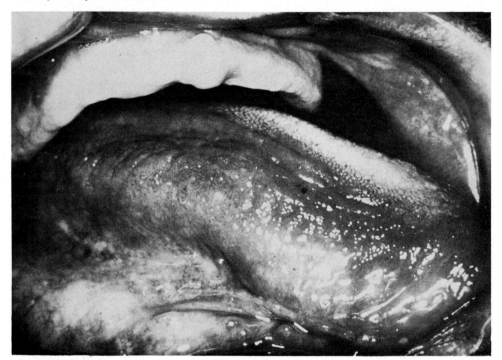

Figure 6.1. Glossitis associated with pernicious anaemia. The dorsum and lateral borders are inflamed, atrophic and ulcerated.

Carbohydrate

Carbohydrate does not constitute an essential nutritional factor, other than for the provision of calories, and accordingly there are no specific general or oral manifestations of deficiency.

Proteins

Once ingested, proteins are broken down into small peptides and amino acids; as such they are absorbed. A number of amino acids, known as essential amino acids, are necessary and are utilized for the synthesis of the body's proteins.

The condition of protein, or amino acid, deficiency is known as kwashiorkor and probably represents a multiple-deficiency state, as a diet which is inadequate in protein is bound to be deficient in other vitamins and minerals.

Patients with kwashiorkor present with glossitis and angular cheilitis, both of which are relatively non-specific oral manifestations of various nutritional deficiencies.

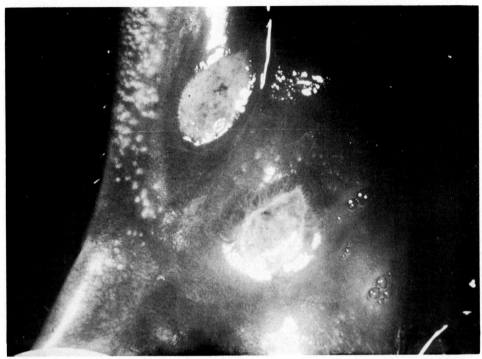

Figure 6.2. Recurrent aphthae in a patient with folate deficiency associated with adult coeliac disease.

Fats

Most lipids can be synthesized in the body. However, two unsaturated fatty acids which are necessary to the diet, linoleic and linolenic acid, cannot be synthesized. These are required in the synthesis of prostaglandins. Although cutaneous changes are well-recognized features of fatty acid deficiency, no mucosal changes have been described.

Vitamins

These will be detailed in the following order:

1. Vitamin A
2. Vitamin B_1 (thiamine)
3. Vitamin B_2 (riboflavin)
4. Vitamin B_6 (pyridoxine)
5. Nicotinic acid (niacin)
6. Pantothenic acid
7. Biotin
8. Vitamin B_{12}
9. Folic acid
10. Vitamin C (ascorbic acid)
11. Vitamin D
12. Vitamin E
13. Vitamin K

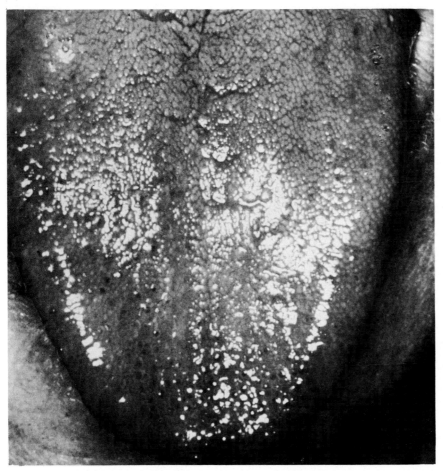

Figure 6.3. Iron deficiency with early atrophic glossitis of tongue tip.

Vitamin A

Vitamin A is a fat soluble vitamin which is necessary for many biological processes, including epithelial proliferation and maturation.

Deficiency of vitamin A may lead to the development of hyperkeratotic white patches on the oral mucosa although no evidence exists to suggest that this deficiency is the cause of the leukoplakia. As the salivary duct epithelium may be similarly affected, there is blockage of saliva with a resultant xerostomia.

An excess of vitamin A, conversely, has been said to lead to epithelial thinning, with red, tender gingivae and scaly lips.

Vitamin B_1 (Thiamine)

There is no convincing evidence that a deficiency of vitamin B_1 leads to the development of any oral symptoms. All vitamins of the B group are water-soluble substances.

Vitamin B₂ (Riboflavin)

Vitamin B$_2$ is utilized for the synthesis of flavoprotein enzymes. Individuals with vitamin B$_2$ deficiency develop angular cheilitis and atrophic glossitis. The fissures at the commissures become infected, with crusting of the surface, and the ulceration may extend along the lips or on to the buccal mucosa.

Vitamin B₆ (Pyridoxine)

Vitamin B$_6$ is necessary for the production of certain co-enzymes.

In cases of vitamin B$_6$ deficiency there is angular cheilitis, atrophic glossitis and ulceration of the mucosa. Peripheral neuritis, which is also a feature of vitamin B$_6$ deficiency, may influence the cranial nerves supplying the oral cavity and signs of nerve degeneration may be evident.

Nicotinic Acid (Niacin)

Nicotinic acid is essential for the synthesis of the two co-enzymes, NAD (nicotinamide-adenine dinucleotide) and NADP (nicotinamide-adenine dinucleotide phosphate). The amount of nicotinic acid needed varies with the level of ingestion of the amino acid, tryptophan, as this can be converted to nicotinic acid.

Nicotinic acid deficiency is termed pellagra and is marked by the three Ds: diarrhoea, dermatitis and dementia. In pellagra, there is atrophic glossitis, oral ulceration and, less commonly, angular cheilitis.

Pantothenic Acid

Although pantothenic acid deficiency has been shown to produce atrophy of the lingual papillae in animals, there is no clear account of this occurring in human beings.

Biotin

There is very little evidence to suggest that biotin deficiency leads to oral changes. The only possible manifestations are of atrophy of the lingual papillae.

Vitamin B₁₂

Vitamin B$_{12}$ interacts with folic acid in the metabolism of pyrimidines and purines, which are necessary for the production of nucleic acids.

Deficiency of vitamin B$_{12}$ is marked by the development of a painful glossitis and oral ulceration, of the aphthous pattern. In the initial stages, there may be only lingual discomfort, but in the later stages of deficiency the tongue takes on a fiery red appearance with, eventually, a smooth shiny surface. Aphthae appear on the non-keratinized oral mucosa as well as on the dorsum of the tongue and it is impossible to differentiate these ulcers clinically from other recurrent aphthae.

Folic Acid

Folic acid is involved in a metabolic process similar to that of vitamin B$_{12}$ and it is hardly surprising that folic acid deficiency has an identical pattern of glossitis and oral ulceration. However, angular cheilitis is another feature of folic acid deficiency: there is doubt as to whether angular cheilitis does or does not develop as a consequence of vitamin B_{12} deficiency.

Vitamin C (Ascorbic Acid)

This is a water-soluble vitamin which is involved in many oxidation reduction reactions. The hallmark of vitamin C deficiency, scurvy, is the development of swollen, ulcerated gingivae which bleed very readily. This reaction is confined to dentate subjects and there is usually a very rapid loss of the supporting alveolar bone, resulting in loosening and eventual shedding of the teeth.

Vitamin D

Vitamin D is a fat-soluble vitamin which is either ingested in the diet or metabolized into an active form in the skin under the effect of ultraviolet radiation. The role of vitamin D is primarily in calcium and bone metabolism and no conclusive changes in the oral mucosa have been ascribed to its deficiency.

Vitamin E

No changes in the oral mucosa have been reported with deficiency of this fat-soluble vitamin.

Vitamin K

Vitamin K, which is another fat-soluble vitamin, is needed for the synthesis of several clotting factors. Accordingly, deficiency of vitamin K is marked by the development of a tendency to bleed.

Mineral

Iron

Iron is a necessary constituent of several enzyme systems, particularly redox reactions.

Iron deficiency is associated with a number of epithelial changes. In the mouth, there is an atrophic glossitis and angular cheilitis. Ulceration of the oral mucosa may also appear and this is clinically the same as aphthae from other causes. The glossitis of iron deficiency is probably not as painful as that associated with vitamin B_{12} and folic acid deficiencies. Less commonly, oral candidosis may be a sign of iron deficiency.

FURTHER READING

Chanarin, I. (1969) in *The Megaloblastic Anaemias.* Oxford: Blackwell.
Ferguson, M. M. (1975) Chapter 5 in Dolby, A. E. (Ed.) *Oral Mucosa in Health and Disease.* Oxford: Blackwell.
Wintrobe, M. M. (1967) *Clinical Hematology.* Philadelphia: Lea & Febiger.

chapter 7

Endocrine Disease

Pituitary
Adrenal Cortex
Thyroid
Parathyroid
Pancreatic Islets
Gonads

The hormonal secretions of the ductless glands permit adaptation to a fluctuating environment by regulating metabolic pathways. Although hormones are often ascribed a specific effect on target tissues it should be appreciated that there is also considerable interaction between the various endocrine glands and, accordingly, any primary abnormality may be accompanied by complex compensatory changes in other glands.

In general, there are no specific local measures for the mouth in the treatment of hormonal disturbances; the management being rectification of the endocrine imbalance.

PITUITARY

The only hormone secreted by the pituitary which possibly has a direct effect upon the oral tissues is somatotropin (growth hormone), although its action may be mediated by the liver. When this is secreted in excess, the abnormalities which subsquently occur depend on the age of the patient, and on whether growth centres are still active; thus general enlargement or gigantism occurs in the child, and acromegaly in the adult. Among the oral changes, the tongue and lips enlarge (Figure 7.1) and the teeth may become spaced as the jaws enlarge. Scalloping may be evident around the lateral margins of the enlarged tongue due to indentations from the dentition.

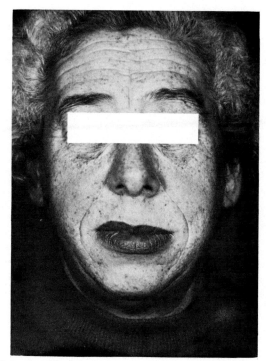

Figure 7.1. Acromegaly: enlargement of lower jaw, lips and supra-orbital ridges.

ADRENAL CORTEX

Addison's disease, or adrenocortical hypofunction, results in a decreased secretion of glucocorticoids, particularly cortisol. The commonest cause of adrenocortical failure is an autoimmune state leading to adrenal atrophy.

Adrenocortical hypofunction is marked by the appearance of brown melanotic pigmentation of the oral mucosa (Figure 7.2). This may occur at any site but is most commonly found on the buccal mucosa. Care must be taken not to mistake physiological pigmentation of the mucosa, a state which is frequently present in dark-skinned races as well as in some Caucasians who have a dark complexion. The clinical appearance may well be identical and if the patient is unsure of the duration of pigmentation further investigations are advisable. Hypoplasia of various endocrine glands, including the adrenal cortex and parathyroids, may be associated with oral candidosis in the endocrine candidosis syndrome.

The opposite condition, an excessive level of corticosteroids, is termed Cushing's syndrome (Figure 7.3). By far the commonest aetiology of this state now is iatrogenic, from the therapeutic administration of steroids.

Candidal infection is a frequent side-effect encountered in patients receiving steroid therapy, especially if the steroids come into direct contact with the oral mucosa as in topical application or during inhalation from nebulizers. The aetiological mechanism of this condition is presumably suppression of the immune response.

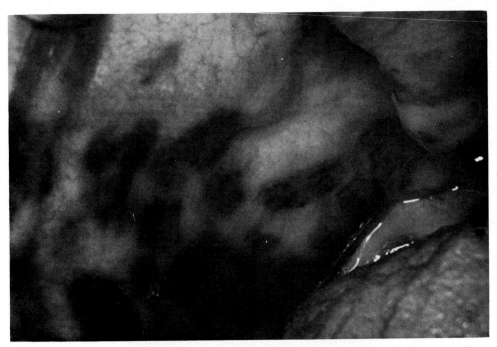

Figure 7.2. Addison's disease, showing early melanin pigmentation of buccal mucosa.

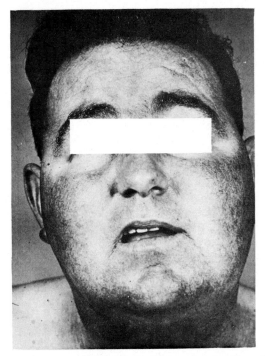

Figure 7.3. Cushing's syndrome due to prolonged steroid drug therapy. Characteristic moon facies and ruddy complexion.

THYROID

A deficiency of thyroxine and tri-iodothyronine, the two thyroid hormones, leads to cretinism in the newborn and myxoedema in adults.

Congenital hypothyroidism is associated with marked enlargement of the tongue which results in its protruding from the mouth. The lips also tend to be puffy and enlarged. Less commonly, the gingivae and palatal mucosa may acquire a spongy appearance. Tooth eruption is also delayed.

In myxoedema, the puffiness of the face and lips is less prominent. No alteration in the oral mucosa itself occurs.

Hyperthyroidism, or thyrotoxicosis, is not associated with any mucosal changes although a tremor of the tongue is sometimes noted.

PARATHYROID

Pathological fluctuations in the levels of parathormone are not responsible for any specific changes in the oral mucosa although candidal infections are common in hypoparathyroidism.

PANCREATIC ISLETS

The B cells of the pancreatic islets secrete insulin. When there is a lack of available insulin for the cells, due either to insufficient production or to inadequate cellular receptors, diabetes mellitus develops.

There are probably no oral manifestations in the well-controlled diabetic, although oral symptoms are often found either during the developmental stages of diabetes mellitus or when it is inadequately controlled, whether the control be with insulin injections, hypoglycaemic drugs or diet alone.

Xerostomia and a marked thirst reflect the polyuria of diabetes. Direct changes also take place in the salivary glands (see Chapter 12). A general burning sensation of the oral tissues may also be indicative of diabetes.

Gingivitis and periodontal disease are more prevalent in poorly controlled diabetics. It is therefore important that all such patients be made conscious of oral hygiene and encouraged to be more enthusiastic than average about it. Unfortunately, the individuals who tend to be careless in the management of their diabetes are also prone to neglect oral hygiene.

Diabetics, again when inadequately controlled, have a lowered resistance to infection and oral candidosis is common. In any patient presenting with candidosis which has no apparent aetiology, it would seem prudent to screen for diabetes mellitus by testing the urine for glucose. In addition, a fasting blood glucose or a glucose tolerance test would be indicated should diabetes be suspected. Cases of recurrent oral candidosis should certainly have this carried out. (For management of candidosis, see Chapter 4.)

Wounds heal more slowly and any ulcers resulting from minor trauma may have a protracted healing period. Oral or facial paraesthesia occasionally occurs as part of the peripheral neuropathy associated with diabetes mellitus.

GONADS

The principal sources of the steroidal sex hormones are the ovaries and testes. The adrenal cortex secretes a small amount and the placenta is a further source during pregnancy.

The actions of sex hormones are complex and it is difficult to obtain a clear impression of their role in oral disease. It does seem, however, that certain oral changes can be associated with an altered hormonal status.

These groups of disorders can be considered under the following headings: periodontal changes, menstrually related aphthae, mucosal changes and the menopause.

Periodontal Changes

The intensity of gingivitis increases during episodes of hormonal fluctuation, namely puberty and pregnancy, possibly in the menstrual cycle and even with ingestion of some oral contraceptives.

The gingivitis and pyogenic granuloma (pregnancy tumour or pregnancy epulis) of pregnancy is well recognized. There seems little doubt that oestrogens and progestogens can influence an inflammatory response and during phases of altered levels the individual is more susceptible to the development of periodontal disease. What in fact occurs is a lowering of the threshold at which an inflammatory reaction will develop in response to plaque. In the presence of good oral hygiene, however, this is not a problem and the only treatment for gingivitis which occurs at puberty or during pregnancy is identical to that at any other time, namely improved oral hygiene.

Whether or not oral contraceptives cause an increase in gingivitis requires further elucidation.

Menstrually Related Aphthae

A small number of females who present with recurrent aphthae give a clear history: the ulcers either appear only in the latter half of the menstrual cycle or are most troublesome at that time. In addition, these ulcers normally clear up within the first trimester of pregnancy only to reappear two or three months after the birth of the child.

Recently, it has been shown that the systemic administration of certain synthetic progestogens may assist patients with this form of ulceration. Consultation with a gynaecologist and with the patient's family doctor is advised before using such treatment.

Mucosal Changes and the Menopause

The menopause is the cessation of menstruation. Women undergoing this phase of profound hormonal change may experience many physical and psychological disorders. On occasion, it may be difficult to decide when the problem is physical or when it is mental, particularly when the patient has symptoms but no apparent clinical signs.

Oral symptoms are fairly common in women during the perimenopausal era and the complaint of a burning sensation in the tongue (glossopyrhosis) is characteristic. There has been considerable speculation as to whether this is a true physical problem or a psychological symptom, but it is difficult to reconcile the constancy of this very specific symptom with general neurotic symptoms: a burning sensation in the mouth is not a regular feature of neurotic or depressed individuals at other ages. It is therefore our belief that this symptom is a physical entity although the aetiology remains to be elucidated. Therapy with oestrogens or progestogens has been disappointing and it remains a most difficult condition to treat.

chapter 8

Haemopoietic Disease

Defective Haemostasis
Anaemia
Polycythaemia
Leucopenia, Neutropenia and Agranulocytosis
Leukaemia

The blood consists of erythrocytes, leucocytes and platelets suspended in plasma. As such, there are several distinct constituents, and disease states exist wherein each of these constituents may be changed either in quantity or quality. Disorders of the blood are relatively common and are frequently associated with changes in the oral mucosa.

It should be appreciated that disorders of the blood may be caused by the same basic underlying defect which is also leading to changes in the oral tissues and the actual alteration in the blood does not in itself produce the oral manifestations. In other instances, however, it is the disorder of the blood which is directly responsible for the signs in the oral tissues.

DEFECTIVE HAEMOSTASIS

Haemostasis is achieved by an initial reflex vasoconstriction followed by the aggregation of platelets. Subsequently, secondary haemostasis is affected by the accumulation of fibrin strands within the clump of platelets, which thus form a plug. Several factors are therefore involved in the attainment of haemostasis following injury and a dysfunction of any may lead to defective haemostasis. The precise sequence of coagulation is complex and the reader is referred to standard textbooks on haematology, e.g. Wintrobe, 1974 (see Further Reading at the end of this chapter).

Disorders of the intravascular haemostatic mechanism may be divided into inadequate platelet function and defective coagulation. Vascular abnormalities only rarely give rise to oral changes.

Platelet Function

Aetiology. Inadequate platelet function is due either to a quantitative deficiency (thrombocytopenia) or to a qualitative deficiency (thromboasthenia and thrombopathia). However, regardless of the actual aetiology of inadequate platelet function, the oral manifestations are the same and these may even represent the initial presentation of the disorder.

Thrombocytopenia is the commonest cause of abnormal bleeding and may be occasioned by numerous aetiological factors (Table 8.1; Figure 8.1).

Table 8.1. *Aetiology of thrombocytopaenia.*

Deficient platelet production
Drug suppression of marrow (e.g. cytotoxic agents, gold compounds, chloramphenicol, phenylbutazone)
Idiopathic aplastic anaemia
Radiation (x-rays and isotopes)
Marrow replacement as in leukaemia and myelofibrosis
Deficiency of vitamin B_{12} and folic acid

Accelerated platelet destruction
Idiopathic thrombocytopenia (autoimmunity)
Drug reactions (e.g. carbamazepine, diphenylhydantoin, methyldopa, sulphathiazole)
Haemolytic anaemia
Systemic lupus erythematosus

Qualitative deficiencies of platelets are rare. In thromboasthenia (Glanzmann's disease) there is diminished clot retraction and platelet aggregation: this condition is inherited as an autosomal recessive trait. Thrombopathia refers to the impaired extrusion of nucleotides, during the release reaction, which disturbs aggregation.

Clinical features. The severity of clinical features is directly related to the diminution of platelets. Spontaneous haemorrhages develop when the platelet count falls below $60 \times 10^9/l$ ($60\,000/\mu l$) and life-endangering haemorrhage is liable to occur with a level below $20 \times 10^9/l$ ($20\,000/\mu l$).

Patients with inadequate platelet function have fine petechial haemorrhages and coarser ecchymoses on the soft palate, floor of the mouth, buccal mucosa and labial mucosa. The gingivae bleed very readily and, with negligible trauma, blood oozes out from the gingival margins. Ill-fitting dentures may be associated with multiple petechiae and minor traumas to the oral mucosa can result in disproportionate bleeding.

Management. The management of individuals with this disorder must, as in all systemic diseases, be directed primarily towards the basic disease. On the other hand, several local measures may be instituted in order to minimize intra-oral bleeding.

Gingivitis promotes the tendency of the gingivae to bleed and a high standard of oral hygiene is essential. During severe phases of inadequate platelet function the teeth should be carefully cleaned, using a medium toothbrush and dental floss. If this causes excessive haemorrhage then it may be necessary to resort to using a 0.2 per cent aqueous chlorhexidine gluconate mouthwash four times daily. Scaling and polishing are reserved for those periods of remission when all dental treatment should be carried out. In the case of teeth with doubtful retention value it is preferable to extract them while the patient possesses a competent haemostatic mechanism rather than to face the risk of an emergency extraction at a more inconvenient phase.

Sources of trauma to the oral mucosa require rectification: ragged edges and sharp cusps should be ground. Ill-fitting dentures are frequently associated with petechiae and therefore must be replaced by new dentures if the occlusal balance or fitting surfaces cannot be corrected.

Dental extractions and other oral surgical procedures are contra-indicated as they can be followed by extremely severe haemorrhage. Should such surgery be imperative, however, the patient must be admitted into hospital and a transfusion of fresh platelets administered. The margins of the socket are routinely sutured, preferably with an absorbable material such as PGA (Dexon). The dentis should consult with the patient's physician before undertaking any treatment likely to cause haemorrhage.

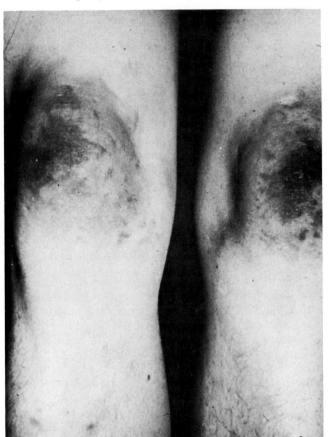

Figure 8.1. Purpura over both knees in a patient with thrombocytopenia.

Blood Coagulation

Aetiology. Haemophilia is defective blood coagulation due to the deficiency of certain clotting factors and this may be either an inherited or an acquired condition (Table 8.2).

Clinical features. Intra-oral bleeding is not as common with haemophilia as it is with inadequate platelet function although petechiae, ecchymoses and severe post-extraction haemorrhage do occur in the more extreme forms of the disorder.

Table 8.2. *Classification of disorders of blood coagulation.*

Platelets
  Thrombocytopenia
  Thromboasthenia

Blood coagulation
(a) Inherited disorders:
  Factor VIII deficiency (haemophilia)
  Factor IX deficiency (Christmas disease)
  Factor XI deficiency
  Factor V deficiency
  Factor VII deficiency
  Factor X deficiency
  Factor XII deficiency
  Von Willebrand's disease
(b) Acquired disorders:
  Deficiency of vitamin K (e.g. drugs such as coumarins; liver disease; deficiency due to malabsorption)
  Accelerated destruction of coagulation factors
  Abnormal inhibitors of coagulation
  Leukaemia
  Multiple myeloma

Management. As with inadequate platelet function, the main local measures are avoidance of extractions and minimization of gingivitis with strict oral hygiene. Again, if a surgical procedure is necessary the patient can be given an infusion of plasma or antihaemophilic globulin, depending on the deficiency. The same operative management of sockets obtains. Patients receiving anticoagulation therapy, such as heparin or warfarin, must be handled with caution and their physician contacted prior to any surgery. Phytamenadione (vitamin K) is a specific antidote to the oral anticoagulants and after intravenous administration acts within 12 to 24 hours.

ANAEMIA

Anaemia is the quantitative or qualitative reduction in erythrocytes which results in a decrease of circulating haemoglobin: the term is applied when the haemoglobin concentration falls below 12.5 g/dl for males and 12.0 g/dl for females. Other than causing pallor of the mucosa, when the haemoglobin level is less than approximately 10 g/dl, anaemia itself does not produce any oral lesion.

Various nutrients for haemoglobin and erythrocyte formation are also essential for a healthy oral mucosa and it is specifically the nutritional deficiencies which produce changes in the mucosa (see Chapter 6). The changes associated with aplastic anaemia are probably attributable to the decreased white cell production.

The accelerated destruction of mature erythrocytes is termed haemolytic anaemia and this may be caused by either intracorpuscular defects or extracorpuscular factors. In patients with severe haemolysis the skin, sclera and oral mucosae become icteric due to hyperbilirubinaemia (Table 8.3).

POLYCYTHAEMIA

Aetiology. Polycythaemia is the abnormal increase in circulating erythrocytes and hence in haemoglobin. It is subdivided into relative polycythaemia, such as occurs in haemoconcentration, primary polycythaemia (polycythaemia vera), and secondary polycythaemia. Polycythaemia vera is a condition of unknown aetiology and the increase in erythrocytes is usually accompanied by increased production of granular leucocytes and platelets, indicating a generalized increase in bone marrow activity. Myelofibrosis or acute leukaemia may eventually develop in these patients.

Secondary polycythaemia develops as a consequence of hypoxia, whatever its cause.

Clinical features. In individuals with polycythaemia the oral mucosa may become a deep red colour with a bluish tinge appearing on the lips. This is due to cyanosis arising from the sluggish circulation of the viscous blood.

Although there is an increased number of platelets, these often have qualitative deficiencies (see section, 'Defective Haemostasis', above) in cases of polycythaemia vera and bleeding of the gingival margins may occur.

Management. Treatment is symptomatic. Haemorrhages around the gums are usually not serious, particularly when the general management involves regular blood letting. Oral hygiene should be strict in order to prevent the development of gingivitis, with its attendant inflammation and greater tendency to bleed from the gingivae.

Table 8.3. *Normal haematological values.*

Haemoglobin:	Male	12.5−17.0 g/dl
	Female	12.0−14.0 g/dl

MCV (mean cell volume): 80−100 fl (80−100 μ^3)

PCV (packed cell volume *or* haematocrit):	Male	42−50%
	Female	38−45%

MCH (mean corpuscular haemoglobin): 27−31 pg

MCHC (mean corpuscular haemoglobin concentration): 32−36 g/dl

Red cell count:	Male	4.5−6.3 × 10^{12}/l (4.5−6.3 million/mm³)
	Female	4.2−5.4 × 10^{12}/l (4.2−5.4 million/mm³)

WBC count: 4.0−10.0 × 10^9/l (4000−10 000/mm³)

Differential WBC count:	neutrophils	60−70%
	lymphocytes	20−53%
	monocytes	2.4−11.8%
	eosinophils	3−8%
	basophils	0.6−1.8%

Platelets: 140−440 × 10^9/l (140 000−440 000/mm³)

LEUCOPENIA, NEUTROPENIA AND AGRANULOCYTOSIS

Aetiology. Leucopenia is, by definition, a fall in the leucocyte cell count below 4.0 × 10^9/l (4000/mm³). The differential white cell count may remain balanced but there is most frequently a disproportionate reduction in the polymorphonuclear neutrophils. In such cases, the term 'neutropenia' is applied. Agranulocytosis represents a very pronounced decrease in the circulating granulocyte series and can be considered as an extreme form of neutropenia. Neutropenia and agranulocytosis may be caused by a broad range of factors including infections, drug ingestion, radiation exposure, leukaemia, myelofibrosis and lymphosarcoma.

In one disorder, a cyclical diminution of polymorphonuclear neutrophils occurs about every three weeks and persists for one week. The aetiology of this cyclic neutropenia is unknown and the periodicity has not been related to any other cyclical variations. During the phase when there is a lowered number of circulating poly-morphonuclear neutrophils, ulceration of the oral mucosa occurs, comparable to that developing in other forms of neutropenia. There is a familial tendency.

Clinical features. The decrease in circulating leucocytes leads to an inability to cope successfully with infections. Although there is individual variation in the level of leucocytes at which oral manifestations initially appear, the lower the white cell count, the greater is the tendency for oral ulceration and gingivitis to develop.

Ulceration may be minimal or it can be extensive, involving the labial, buccal, palatal, gingival and pharyngeal mucosae. The ulcers become deep, often with ragged margins, infected and covered with a yellowish-grey slough. These cause considerable distress and interfere with eating.

Management. The detailed management of this extensive oral ulceration is discussed below (see 'Leukaemia — Ulceration and Infection'); the essential steps being relief of pain, control of infection and preventive measures.

LEUKAEMIA

Leukaemia is a disease of unknown aetiology characterized by the abnormal and excessive proliferation of the leucocyte precursors and is usually associated with an increase in the number of circulating leucocytes. Both acute and chronic forms of leukaemia exist and these can be further subdivided into lymphocytic, myelocytic and monocytic variants. All age groups may be affected although the acute forms are commoner in younger people and chronic leukaemia occurs more often in the over-20s age group.

Clinical features. In different reported series, oral complications of leukaemia range from 13 to 87 per cent of patients. Acute leukaemia is associated with the greater incidence of oral changes, being about three times as great as in chronic leukaemia. Of these acute leukaemias, the myelocytic and monocytic variants have the most frequent and severe oral changes. The oral manifestations are mucosal pallor, petechiae and ecchymoses, gingivitis and gingival bleeding, ulceration, gingival hypertrophy and infections (Figure 8.2).

Although the precise frequency of oral manifestations is disputed, these lesions within the mouth constitute one of the greatest sources of discomfort to the patient and may lead to a decreased intake of food and even of fluids. Furthermore, the chemo-therapeutic agents which are employed in the management of leukaemia can themselves induce ulcerative stomatitis; these include methotrexate (amethopterin), cyclo-phosphamide, daunorubicin, 6-mercaptopurine, cytosine arabinoside and chlor-ambucil. Corticosteroids depress the immune response and so promote the development of secondary infections. Leukaemia is a hazard to life and a physician or clinical haematologist will undertake the patient's overall care.

Mucosal Pallor

When the haemoglobin falls to below 10 g/dl the mucous membranes become pale in colour. The anaemia is caused by haemorrhagic losses together with decreased erythropoiesis due to replacement of the bone marrow with the diseased tissue.

There are no oral symptoms attributable to the mucosal pallor per se and accordingly no local treatment is required.

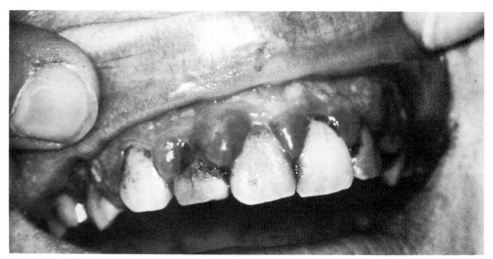

Figure 8.2. Gingivitis and gingival hypertrophy in a patient with monocytic leukaemia.

Petechiae and Ecchymoses: Gingival Bleeding

A haemorrhagic tendency is the most common oral manifestation of leukaemia. This is caused mainly by a reduction in platelets as well as, to a lesser extent, disordered coagulation and more active fibrinolysis.

The oral changes associated with defective haemostasis and their management are detailed above (in 'Defective Haemostasis'; and see Figure 8.3).

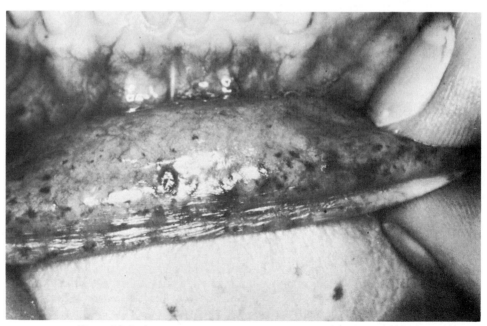

Figure 8.3. Ecchymoses, due to thrombocytopenia, in a leukaemic patient.

Gingivitis

Gingivitis and periodontal disease are other common findings in leukaemic patients with an apparent increase in the gingival tissues as a reaction to plaque accumulation. Once gingivitis is established, normal oral hygiene tends to decline further because of the discomfort caused by brushing. In addition, these individuals are often most unwell and therefore incapable of cleaning their teeth effectively.

Any patient diagnosed as having leukaemia requires oral hygiene instruction as well as long-term enthusiastic supervision. Gingivitis in leukaemia can often be controlled if the oral hygiene is of a sufficiently high standard.

Should a patient not be fit enough to clean his own teeth adequately, an electric toothbrush is most useful and is also more readily employed by a nurse. A dental gel containing 1 per cent chlorhexidine (Corsodyl, ICI) has recently become available and would seem to be a useful adjunct to toothpaste. In addition to brushing, a mouth-rinse of 0.2 per cent aqueous chlorhexidine gluconate four times daily inhibits plaque formation and can be used either in conjunction with or as a substitute for brushing.

Ulceration and Infection

Ulceration of the oral mucosa in leukaemia probably has a multi-factorial aetiology. In some instances, the capillaries and arterioles are completely occluded by emboli of leukaemic cells and so cause the overlying mucosa to become gangrenous and to slough.

Hypogammaglobulinaemia and granulocytopenia are common in leukaemia and hence there is a decreased ability to cope with infections. Extensive oral ulceration develops with large, ragged, infected ulcers appearing on the labial, buccal, palatal, lingual, gingival and pharyngeal mucosae; a multitude of organisms may be associated with these ulcers (Figure 8.4). In addition, folate deficiency is known to produce oral ulceration, and methotrexate, a commonly used folic acid antagonist in the management of acute leukaemia, has been shown to have ulcer-inducing potential. In these circumstances, the topical use of folinic acid, in the form of calcium leucovorin mouthwash, is of considerable value. As has been mentioned above, several other chemotherapeutic agents which are also used to treat leukaemia may cause oral ulceration due to their disturbance of the normal dynamic equilibrium of cell division and maturation.

Where oral ulceration is present, it is essential that the teeth are routinely examined in order that any sharp edges may be thoroughly smoothed. In the edentulous, dentures must be well-fitting and occlusally balanced for minimal mucosal irritation. Use of a soft-base liner is a suitable temporary measure for loose-fitting dentures.

The use of a zinc sulphate mouthwash six times daily relieves much of the discomfort of ulceration as well as apparently promoting healing. In cases where ulceration is widespread and pain is severe enough to inhibit eating, the patient is given 5 ml of a 2 per cent topical lignocaine hydrochloride preparation (Xylocaine Viscous Solution or Xylotox Oral) to hold in the mouth for two minutes prior to meals: with large ulcers, the use of 4 per cent lignocaine paste or cream will afford considerable relief.

Cracked and bleeding lips often accompany oral ulceration and this complication may be alleviated by the regular application of petroleum jelly or lanolin cream.

Dental extractions and surgical procedures within the mouth are to be avoided if at all possible since not only is there the immediate problem of haemorrhage but cellulitis and osteomyelitis may readily ensue.

The incidence and severity of bacterial infections in leukaemia are related to the degree of granulocytopenia. Suspect lesions should have swabs taken for routine microbiological investigation. Mucosal infections respond well to regular mouth-washing with 0.2 per cent aqueous chlorhexidine solution, every two hours throughout the day. An alternative antiseptic mouthwash is 0.5 to 1.0 per cent povidone-iodine (Betadine) and this has the slight theoretical advantage of also being effective against *Pseudomonas*.

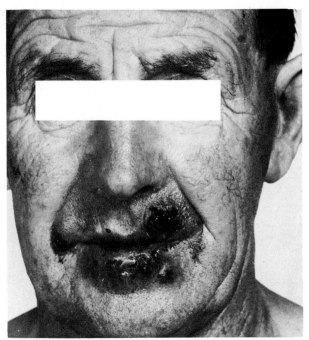

Figure 8.4. Perioral ulceration due to herpes simplex infection in a patient receiving cytotoxic drugs for chronic lymphatic leukaemia.

Candidal infection is frequently found superimposed on oral ulceration in addition to existing solely as a surface infection. After isolation and identification of the fungus, amphotericin B lozenges or nystatin lozenges, to be sucked four times daily, are normally prescribed. For severely debilitated patients a suspension of amphotericin B or natamycin is available; several drops of this can be run into the mouth at regular intervals.

Should there be a candidal infection with angular cheilitis, amphotericin B or nystatin ointment should be applied four times daily. The more recently introduced miconazole cream (Daktarin) has the additional advantages of being active against certain gram-positive cocci as well as fungi and is therefore a particularly suitable preparation for mixed infections.

If the patient is edentulous, dentures should be removed after every meal and scrubbed in running water; overnight they must be removed and stored in a 1 per cent sodium hypochlorite (Milton) or a 2 per cent chlorhexidine solution. The dentures must be thoroughly rinsed before insertion. The most convenient time to administer the antifungal lozenge is when the dentures are out for cleaning, thus enabling the drug to reach the entire mucosa. A thin smear of miconazole, amphotericin B or nystatin cream should be applied to the fitting surfaces of the dentures prior to re-insertion as candida proliferates particularly actively under dentures.

Gingival hypertrophy

Gingival hypertrophy is a particular feature of the monocytic and myelocytic forms of leukaemia and is very rarely seen in lymphocytic leukaemia. The gross enlargement may virtually engulf the teeth and this is due to a dense leucocyte infiltrate which disrupts the normal connective tissue morphology.

This hypertrophy is difficult to treat and gingivectomy is obviously contra-indicated. Our approach has been to maintain optimal oral hygiene together with the use of frequent hot salt mouthwashes. A periodontal pack may be of value to some patients but it is doubtful whether the discomfort and difficulty of applying this is usually worth while. Any cusps of opposing teeth which are traumatizing areas of hypertrophied gingiva should be ground down.

FURTHER READING

General

Ferguson, M. M. (1975) Chapter 5 in Dalby, A. E. (Ed.) *The Oral Mucosa in Health and Disease.* Oxford: Blackwell Scientific Publications.
Wintrobe, M. M. (1974) *Clinical Haematology.* Philadelphia: Lea & Febiger.

Leukaemia

Bodey, G. P. (1971) Oral complications of the myeloproliferative diseases. *Postgraduate Medical Journal,* **69,** 115.
Ferguson, M. M., Dagg, J. H., Hunter, I. P. & Stephen, K. W. (1978) The presentation and management of oral lesions in leukaemia. *Journal of Dentistry* (in press).
Lynch, M. A. & Ship, I. I. (1967) Oral manifestations of leukemia: a postdiagnostic study. *Journal of the American Dental Association,* **75,** 1139-1144.

Haemostasis

Linenberg, W. B. (1964) Idiopathic thrombocytopenic purpura. *Oral Surgery, Oral Medicine and Oral Pathology,* **17,** 22-29.

Cardiovascular Disease

CYANOSIS

Cyanosis is the term used to describe the bluish colour of the mucous membranes and skin which results from an increase in the amount of reduced haemoglobin in the superficial vessels. Once the quantity of reduced haemoglobin exceeds 5 g/dl, cyanosis usually becomes apparent and it is important to appreciate that cyanosis depends upon an absolute value, rather than on a relative amount, of reduced haemoglobin. Accordingly, cyanosis does not occur in severe anaemia, where the total haemoglobin falls below 5 g/dl.

Cyanosis is divided into *central* and *peripheral* cyanosis. Central cyanosis is due to a decreased oxygen saturation such as is caused by impaired pulmonary function or veno-arterial shunts, e.g. congenital heart disease. In central cyanosis, the oral mucosa and lips, as well as the cheeks, ears and nail beds, may appear blue. However, the circulation is adequate and the peripheries are warm.

Peripheral cyanosis arises when the blood flow is sluggish, such as in vasoconstriction and vascular obstruction, and the reduced oxygen tension within the capillaries results in the bluish coloration. In contrast to central cyanosis, the peripheries are cold in peripheral cyanosis and the lips and oral mucosa are rarely affected.

ATHEROSCLEROSIS

Atherosclerosis is the most common disease of the arteries in adults and is characterized by the deposition of lipids in a patchy or irregular fashion in the deeper layers of the intima. The disease affects large- and medium-sized arteries and produces narrowing of the vessel lumen or weakness of its wall. Occlusion may occur, particularly when there is superimposed thrombosis. Atherosclerosis of the coronary arteries is an important and common cause of ischaemic heart disease (see below) but the disease also affects other arterial systems such as those supplying the oral structures. It may result in a gradual failure of the blood supply through the inferior dental system.

There is no convincing evidence that the altered blood supply due to atherosclerosis is a factor in causing periodontal or other oral disease, but it has been suggested that it may reduce the local resistance to injurious agents or the ability for repair following injury in middle or old age.

TEMPORAL ARTERITIS

Temporal arteritis is a disease of the elderly in which the temporal artery, and sometimes other cranial arteries and the aorta and its larger branches, are involved in an inflammatory process characterized by the appearance of giant cells in the media. The lumen is narrowed and there may be associated thrombosis. Women are more often affected than men, and pain is the outstanding symptom. Headache, neck stiffness, pain on talking or chewing or pain in the tongue are likely symptoms, and anorexia weight loss, vague aches and pains and visual symptoms are common.

The superficial temporal arteries are found to be nodular and tender and they may lack pulsation. Usually, the erythrocyte sedimentation rate is elevated above 40 mm in one hour and the patient is febrile.

Blindness and other ill effects may result from this disease. Early diagnosis is important and prompt institution of corticosteroid therapy reduces the likelihood of serious complication. In mild cases, the disease tends to reduce in activity over a period of months or years. The disease is of importance in dentistry as a cause of facial or oral pain but confirmation of the diagnosis and treatment is a matter for the physician.

CORONARY ARTERY DISEASE

Coronary artery disease is usually atherosclerotic in nature and, as indicated above, is an important cause of morbidity and mortality in men older than 40 years of age and in women older than 50. Younger patients are affected less frequently. Narrowing of a coronary artery may cause pain on exertion whereas occlusion tends to cause continuous pain. The pain is usually experienced substernally in the chest, but about one patient in 10 with the disease gives a site other than the chest as the primary location of pain. The jaws and teeth are the only site of a toothache-like pain in a minority of patients; but this pain may also be experienced in the tongue or palate. When a cardiac pain affects sites removed from the heart, it usually does so in company with more typical pain in the chest, shoulder, arm or wrist and there may be a history relating the pain to physical effort, emotional tension, and large meals or exposure to a cold atmosphere. In particular, anginal pain is reduced by rest and by nitroglycerin, though the pain of occlusion may persist.

Some patients regard any symptom presenting outside the mouth as outside the competence of the dentist and may fail to report symptoms such as chest pain unless specifically asked: 'Does the pain radiate elsewhere or affect any other part of the body?' Pain due to coronary artery disease should be considered in the differential diagnosis of jaw pain when no local cause is apparent. Confirmation of the diagnosis and treatment of the disease is a matter for the physician.

THE RISK OF INFECTIVE ENDOCARDITIS

It is considered that patients who have thickening of the cusps of the heart valves due to rheumatic or other heart disease, or who have congenital heart disease, are more likely to develop infective endocarditis following bacteraemia than are others who do not have these abnormalities. Patients who have had cardiac surgery are also at risk in this way. Manipulations in the mouth, such as tooth extraction, subgingival sealing or root filling, cause bacteraemia and it seems reasonable to protect patients who suffer from the diseases referred to above by antibiotic cover during the period of risk. Infective endocarditis, although it is uncommon, will cause further damage to the heart and even death, should it occur, and its diagnosis is a matter of some difficulty. Thus, prevention is preferable to the disease even when that prevention carries with it the small hazard associated with antibiotic administration.

Patients who are considered to be susceptible to the risk of infective endocarditis are given 'antibiotic cover' if they are to be subjected to any procedure likely to cause a bacteraemia. The antibiotic should be given so that its maximum concentration in the blood coincides with the operation. The standard procedure is to give 1×10^6 units of benzylpenicillin along with 500 mg streptomycin intramuscularly 30 minutes prior to extraction and phenoxymethylpenicillin by mouth for three days thereafter, in doses of 250 mg every six hours. For patients known to be, or suspected of being, allergic to penicillin, or who have received penicillin within the previous six weeks, erythromycin is a satisfactory alternative. This should be given as 100 mg erythromycin ethylsuccinate by intramuscular injection 30 minutes prior to the operation and by mouth in doses of 250 mg every six hours for three days thereafter. The doses given above are appropriate for adults and should be modified for children. Patients who require protection as above should be advised to report to a physician should they develop a fever or become unwell in the mouth following the dental operation.

Infective endocarditis may occur in the normal heart and the risk of this disease is not necessarily related to the degree of previous damage to the heart: indeed, quite mild cardiac defects may be complicated by infective endocarditis, which may be the first indication that such a defect is present. Patients with rheumatic valvular disease are also often placed on long-term penicillin therapy to prevent the opportunity of reactivation of the rheumatic process and, as stated above, such patients should receive an antibiotic other than penicillin for preventive purposes, since the strains of bacteria in their mouths which will cause bacteraemia are likely to be penicillin resistant.

chapter 10

Dermatological Disease

Inherited Diseases Causing White Lesions on the Oral Mucosa
Inherited Diseases Causing Bullae in the Mouth
Inherited Disorders which Chiefly Affect the Dermis
Acquired Skin Diseases which have Oral Manifestations
Acquired Skin Diseases with Oral Manifestations Characterized by Bulla Formation
Collagen Diseases Affecting the Skin and Mucous Membranes

Many diseases of the skin also affect the oral mucosa and it is convenient to consider these as a group. No satisfactory classification of these diseases exists: lack of knowledge of the cause of some precludes a classification based on aetiology, and their separation on clinical appearances is difficult because a number of them have a variety of clinical forms. The classification used below is based on our present knowledge of aetiology and on certain clinical and histological features.

INHERITED DISEASES CAUSING WHITE LESIONS ON THE ORAL MUCOSA

White Sponge Naevus

This uncommon condition may be present at birth or may appear shortly after, or in childhood or adolescence. It presents in the mouth as white patches which are often widespread, involving the gingiva and cheeks and elsewhere appearing as thickened, spongy, folded lesions (Figure 10.1). Similar patches often occur on other mucosal surfaces. The disease is inherited as an autosomal dominant trait but a familial pattern may be discovered only when all the members of the family are examined since the condition may pass unnoticed or be accepted as 'normal' in a family accustomed to its occurrence.

Histology is helpful in diagnosis: the acanthotic epithelium shows very marked parakeratosis and is remarkable for the intracellular oedema of the cells in the prickle cell and cornified layers.

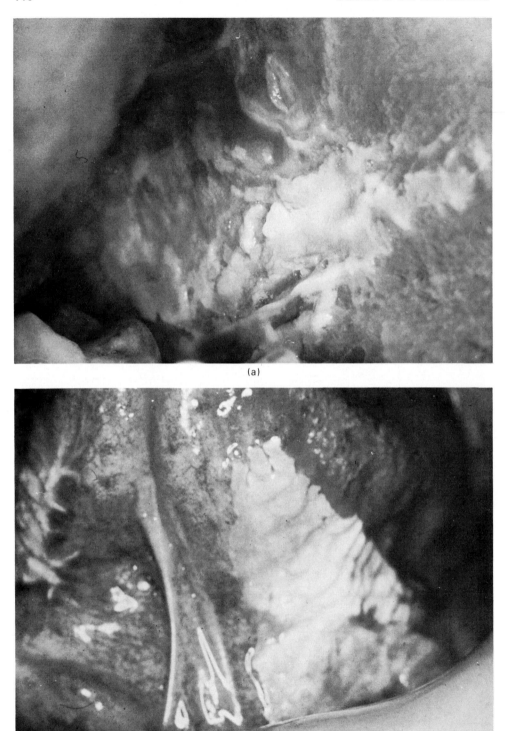

(a)

(b)

Figure 10.1. White sponge naevus: (a) raised irregular white patches on buccal mucosa; (b) wrinkled white patch on ventral surface of tongue (similar lesion on R side has been excised).

Once the diagnosis has been established, no treatment is given because the disease has no ill effects. However, this comment excludes the lesion previously described by some as an epithelial naevus which appeared in adults as an evenly distributed bilateral white patch, sometimes folded or thickened, on the floor of the mouth: such white patches are best regarded as leukoplakic in character and require the careful assessment and management accorded to all leukoplakias.

Pachyonychia Congenita

The oral white patches are histologically reminiscent of white sponge naevus but dystrophic changes in the finger and toe nails, palmar and plantar hyperkeratosis, and excessive sweating also occur in this uncommon inherited disease. Other signs include corneal dystrophy and thickening of the laryngeal, nasal, and tympanic lining epithelium. The condition is associated with a favourable prognosis.

Dyskeratosis Congenita

It is most important that this rare condition be distinguished from the two diseases mentioned above because of the likelihood of malignant transformation of the oral lesions. The disease is inherited and is characterized by oral leukoplakia, dystrophic changes of the nails and pigmentation of the skin. Histologically, the condition resembles leukoplakia with hyperkeratosis and with a focal cellular atypia which increases in severity as the disease progresses. The oral lesions appear before, or in early, adolescence and deteriorate relentlessly until malignancy supervenes in the fourth or fifth decades.

Darier's Disease (Keratosis Follicularis)

This uncommon inherited disorder is dominated by skin lesions, red papules which eventually ulcerate and crust. They tend to occur in the upper part of the body at first but are eventually widespread. Whitish rough papules are also found on the mucosa in many cases. The histology is helpful in diagnosis, but the patient is unlikely to seek treatment from a dentist in the first instance.

INHERITED DISEASES CAUSING BULLAE IN THE MOUTH

Epidermolysis Bullosa

This is an uncommon disease of the skin which exists in five different forms, each with distinctive features. There are simple and dystrophic forms inherited as autosomal dominant characteristics, in which oral bullae occur in a minority of cases and the teeth are not affected. Both forms are dominated by the skin bullae. Further dystrophic and lethal forms are inherited as autosomal recessive characteristics and the former is best known for its oral manifestations. The latter results in early death of the infant. Finally, there is a rare acquired form which does not appear to be inherited.

The dystrophic recessive form appears shortly after birth, with the appearance of bullae after minor trauma to the skin or without apparent cause. The bullae can be initiated by firmly stroking the skin (Nikolsky's sign) and, on rupturing, they leave a painful erosion which heals with scar formation. Ultimately the fingers are destroyed as functioning units and the hands become unsightly and club-shaped (Figure 10.2).

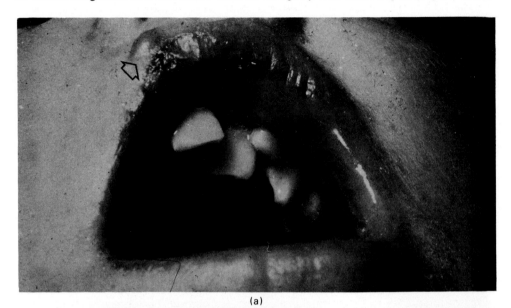

(a)

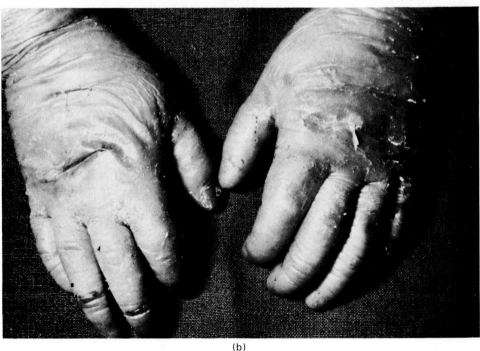

(b)

Figure 10.2. Epidermolysis bullosa: (a) bulla on upper lip; (b) hands of same patient showing extensive involvement and ruptured bullae.

Oral bullae occur after minor trauma and leave painful erosions, with healing by scarification, as on the skin. The result is difficulty in eating, speaking and talking as the scar tissue formed within the mouth limits movement of the lips, tongue and other oropharyngeal structures. The teeth may be absent or malformed in some cases. The bullae tend to be subepidermal in type.

Benign Familial Chronic Pemphigus

This disease is transmitted as a dominant characteristic, though with inconstant effect. Its importance lies in the differential diagnosis of pemphigus vulgaris which it resembles histologically as an intra-epithelial acantholytic bullous disease. However, a familial pattern of occurrence, the appearance of the disease in young adults, and the distribution and appearance of the skin lesions (chiefly on skin exposed to friction and showing a tendency to peripheral extension with central healing) help to differentiate the two.

INHERITED DISORDERS WHICH CHIEFLY AFFECT THE DERMIS

Ehlers—Danlos Syndrome

This is a rare disease which affects the skin and other tissues in the body but which has relatively minor oral manifestations. The disease is inherited, usually as a dominant characteristic, and is present throughout life. The outstanding sign is the unusual elasticity and fragility of the skin. Bruising occurs easily and skin wounds are slow to heal. The tendency to bruising is apparent within the mouth and gingival bleeding may occur. Hyperelasticity of the oral mucosa may not be apparent, although hypermobility of the temporomandibular joints occurs, in common with other joints. Histologically, there is a reduction in the amount of collagen in the skin and its structure is abnormal. The elastic tissue is increased in quantity. The dentine of the teeth is malformed, as is to be expected in a disease which affects mesodermally derived structures.

ACQUIRED SKIN DISEASES WHICH HAVE ORAL MANIFESTATIONS

Erythema Multiforme

This term describes a group of symptoms and signs with multifactorial aetiology. The disease affects the skin and the mucous membrane and appears abruptly, usually in young adult males, although other ages and females may be affected. The cause of the disease is unknown but the deposition of immune complexes, the antigen being microbial in origin or associated with certain drugs, is suspected of being involved in its production. Viral infections, such as herpes simplex, and the use of drugs, such as barbiturates, have been implicated in some cases, although many stimuli appear able to 'trigger' this acute mucocutaneous reaction.

The skin lesions have many forms, macular, papular, vesicular, or bullous, and chiefly affect the extremities (upper and lower limbs, face and neck). Sometimes they have a 'target' or 'iris' appearance composed of concentric rings of varying erythema or oedema. The oral mucosa is often extensively involved and erythematous patches pass quickly through a bullous phase to erosion as the mucous membrane forming the roof of the bulla becomes necrotic. Typically, when the patient is seen, there are bloody encrustations on extensive labial erosions and other eroded areas are present in the mouth and pharynx; the patient complains of pain and proper examination of the mouth is difficult because of the blood-encrusted painful lips (Figure 10.3). The patient is often pyrexic in the early stages of the disease, but the disease tends to be self-limiting, with healing occurring in three or four weeks. Recurrence may be triggered by re-exposure to the causative stimulus. When the disease occurs in a severe form it is described as the Stevens—Johnson syndrome and the patient may be so ill that he requires careful medical supervision in hospital. The conjunctiva and genital mucosa may be involved.

Histologically, in the early stages, changes are found around the superficial blood vessels as perivascular mononuclear cell cuffing. Later, subepithelial and intra-epithelial bullae develop and there is necrosis of the whole thickness of the epithelium, resulting in the erosions seen clinically. In mild cases, the treatment is aimed at reducing the discomfort suffered by the patient. Extensive oral involvement may call for the use of an antiseptic mouthwash. In severely ill patients, antibiotics may be required to prevent secondary respiratory tract infection and systemic administration of steroids results in improvement. However, such severely ill patients need careful medical supervision and their treatment is best given by a dermatologist or physician.

Lichen Planus

This is a disease which involves the skin and the mucous membranes; the involvement of the latter preceding the former sufficiently often to warrant an interest in the disease by dentists. The disease is also important as a differential diagnosis of leukoplakia.

The cause of lichen planus is unknown, although exposure to stress has been implicated in some cases. Patients with the disease are said to be perfectionist in daily living, constantly striving to maintain a high standard in their work and personal lives which may cause symptoms of stress when they are frustrated in achieving the ideal they have projected for themselves. Nevertheless, the clinician should be warned against instant psychiatric diagnosis; psychiatric diagnosis is properly the concern of those trained in that discipline.

In other patients, the disease may follow the ingestion of certain drugs. Gold, arsenicals, streptomycin, PAS, and some anti-malarial and anti-rheumatic drugs have been implicated occasionally in this respect. Those cases of lichen planus which are drug-induced are sometimes described as 'lichenoid eruptions' although this distinction would seem to be unwarranted until there is a proper understanding of the pathogenesis of the disease. It has been suggested that the epithelial change which occurs in lichen planus is the result of lymphocytic activity beneath the epithelium, perhaps representing an immune response to host antigens altered by some unrecognized stimulus. Some reports have described a greater than expected frequency of diabetes among patients with the disease but the relationship, if any, between the two is imperfectly understood at present.

The disease tends to affect adults, and women slightly more often than men. Often, it has an insidious onset and the patient will be unable to date the first appearance of the oral lesions. Intense itching is associated with the skin lesions (Figure 10.4) but the oral lesions may be found, unexpectedly, on routine examination by the dental practitioner or noticed by the patient after casual self-examination to uncover the cause of mild roughness (Figure 10.5).

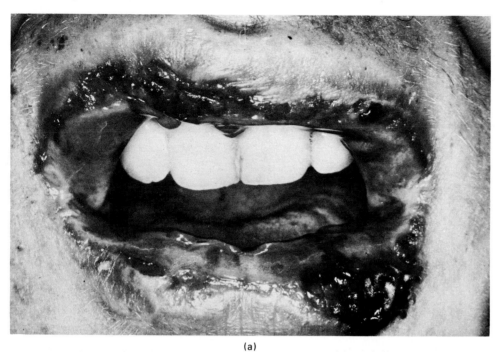

(a)

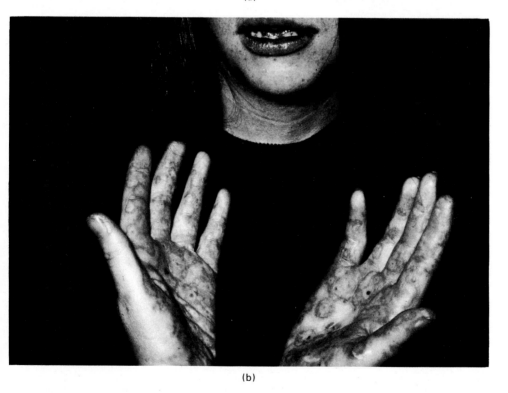

(b)

Figure 10.3. Erythema multiforme: (a) extensive oral ulceration and crusting of lips; (b) characteristic target lesions on skin.

The skin lesions are papular in form and occur most frequently on the flexor surfaces of the arms and inner surfaces of the legs, although the trunk and genitalia may also be affected. The lesions are red or purple with fine white lines, 'Wickham's striae', which may be observed only through a hand lens, on their surface.

The oral lesions are found most frequently on the buccal mucous membrane but also often on the tongue. The lips, gingiva, floor of mouth and palate are less frequently

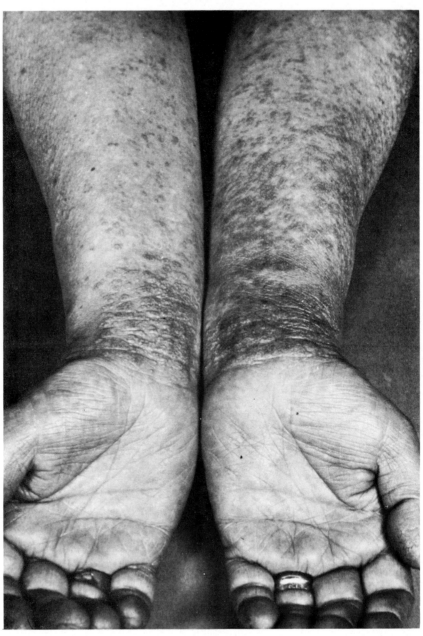

(a)

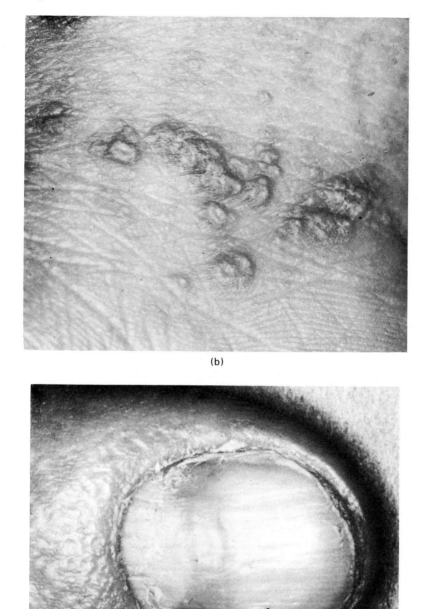

(b)

(c)

Figure 10.4. Lichen planus, skin manifestations: (a) flexor surfaces of wrist and forearms; (b) close up of papular rash; (c) linear ridging of finger nail (arrowed) and papular rash on adjacent skin.

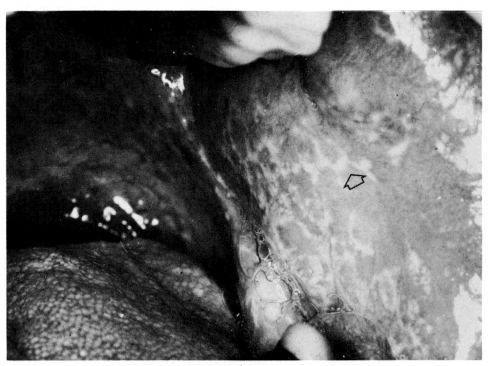

(a)

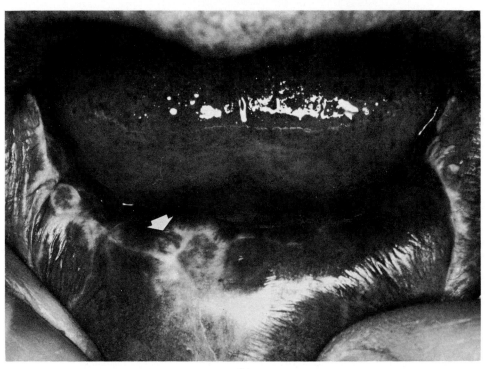

(b)

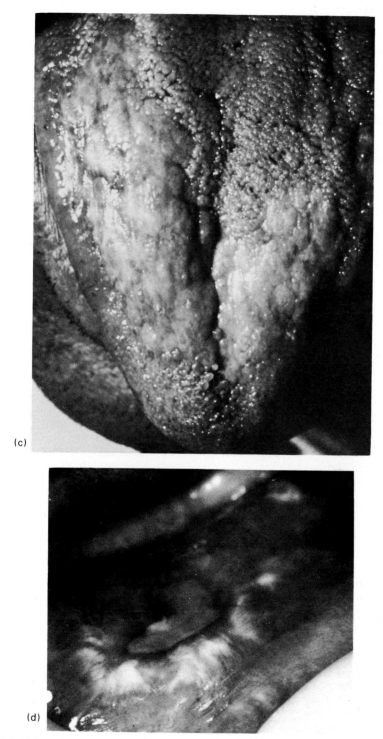

(c)

(d)

Figure 10.5. Lichen planus, oral manifestations: (a) buccal mucosa, reticular pattern; (b) labial mucosa, linear and plaque pattern; (c) lingual mucosa, plaque pattern; (d) labial mucosa, erosive type.

involved. The oral lesions appear as white or grey-white papules, usually linear and sometimes forming complex lace-like or spider-net patterns. Less frequently, the papules are rounded or coalesce to form plaque-like lesions. The latter may have the more typical linear pattern radiating from their periphery.

Although bullae are rarely seen there is an erosive variety in which the epithelium has been stripped away leaving the corium covered by a layer of yellowish fibrin. This erosive variety is painful, particularly when the tongue or commissural regions are affected.

Histological examination of non-erosive lichen planus reveals changes which often vary in degree from place to place in the section under examination, commensurate with the linear appearance seen clinically. There is hyperparakeratosis, or hyperorthokeratosis with a prominent granular cell layer; acanthosis, sometimes producing the sharp-pointed elongated rete ridges described as a 'sawtooth' appearance; liquefactive degeneration of the basal cell layer which varies in degree and which by differentially affecting surfaces of the rete ridges produces the 'sawtooth' appearance described above; and a dense band of lymphocytes immediately beneath the epithelium.

Lichen planus, a chronic disease, may persist for months or years. Its clinical appearance usually permits its differentiation from leukoplakia, but biopsy should be undertaken where there is doubt. Lichen planus is usually a non-malignant condition but malignant change may occur, infrequently, particularly in long-standing erosive or plaque-like forms of the disease. For this reason long-term review of the oral lesions is recommended.

Treatment of the disease is largely ineffective. An attempt should be made to uncover an underlying cause, such as was given above, and relief may follow exclusion of this. Every effort should be made to encourage healing in erosive lichen planus by removing possible local sources of trauma or irritation, by use of an antibacterial mouthwash if the erosions are superficially infected and by corticosteroid preparations applied topically. Useful preparations include hydrocortisone lozenges B.P.C. (Corlan Pellets), Triamcinolone Dental Paste, B.P.C. (Adcortyl in Orabase) and betamethasone 17-valerate pellets, each containing 0.1 mg of the active principle. Apparent exacerbations of the disease may be due to secondary infection with *Candida albicans* which will require appropriate treatment.

Psoriasis

This is a common dermatological disorder and in European skin clinics is seen more frequently than the other diseases referred to in this section. The disease persists for a long time but the mouth is affected only infrequently.

Psoriasis usually appears in the second or third decades of life, with equal frequency in males and females, as small erythematous papules which gradually spread to involve more and more skin. The papules are covered by a thin scale and removal of this reveals a red surface with tiny bleeding points. There is no pain or pruritis and the extent of involvement is variable. The elbows and knees are often affected; the hands and feet seldom. The disease is characterized by periods of exacerbation and remission and a significant number of patients who have it develop arthritis.

Oral lesions occur infrequently but, when they do, may be associated with exacerbation of the skin disease. They appear as erythematous, or greyish, slightly raised plaque or papules, varying in size from a few to several millimetres. Scaling is sometimes noted, as in the skin lesions, and focal ulceration may occur. Considerable caution is advised in assessing oral lesions in patients with psoriasis, since one would expect common oral diseases to occur by chance in patients with this common skin disease and the association of a particular oral lesion with psoriasis in a patient is not proof of a common basis for the skin and mucous membrane lesions.

Histologically, psoriasis is characterized by parakeratosis, microabscesses in the superficial layers of the epithelium, elongation and clubbing of the rete ridges and extension of highly vascular dermal papillae superficially into the epidermis to give the bleeding points which are noted clinically when the scale is removed.

ACQUIRED SKIN DISEASES WITH ORAL MANIFESTATIONS CHARACTERIZED BY BULLA FORMATION

The diseases to be included in this section are classified according to the level of blister formation (Table 10.1). The term bulla is used to describe a blister of appreciable size whereas vesicle describes a blister only a few millimetres in diameter. These diseases fall into two major groups. In the first, the blister forms within the epithelium, either by a loss of attachment between individual epithelial cells (acantholysis) as in pemphigus and familial benign chronic pemphigus, or by oedema within the epithelium and epithelial cell destruction, as in certain viral infections (see Chapter 4). In the second major group, the blister formation takes place as a result of separation of the whole epithelium from the corium as in benign mucous membrane pemphigoid and bullous pemphigoid. Several of the diseases listed in Table 10.1 have received attention in other sections and the reader is referred to these sections for a full account of them.

Table 10.1. *Oral vesiculo-bullous diseases.*

Intra-epithelial	
Acantholytic:	pemphigus
	familial benign chronic pemphigus
Viral:	herpes simplex, etc.
Subepithelial	
	benign mucous membrane pemphigoid
	bullous pemphigoid
	dermatitis herpetiformis
	lichen planus
	epidermolysis bullosa
	erythema multiforme

Pemphigus

This is an uncommon disease characterized by extensive bullae, which rupture to leave erosions, on the oral mucous membrane and skin; the former often appearing as the first manifestation of the disease. In the pre-corticosteroid era the disease carried a high mortality rate but treatment with steroid preparations has markedly improved the situation, although early diagnosis with rapid control of the disease assists in achieving a satisfactory outcome.

In pemphigus a raised titre of antibodies, chiefly IgG in type, to the intercellular substance of the epithelium can be detected using the fluorescent antibody technique. These antibodies appear to be specific for intercellular substance. The disease probably represents an autoreaction to intercellular material, the antibody production being stimulated by some antigenic substance cross-reactive with intercellular material.

However, the pathogenesis of the disease is not fully understood at present.

Several forms of pemphigus are recognized but oral lesions occur in only two:

1. Pemphigus vulgaris
2. Pemphigus vegetans

Pemphigus vulgaris occurs chiefly in patients of 40 years and over, affects the Jewish race more frequently than other races, and males and females equally. The disease may progress rapidly or there may be several weeks or months between the initial presentation and widespread involvement of the skin and mucous membranes.

The skin blisters tend at first to be localized to one part but eventually they occur in sizes varying from a few millimetres to several centimetres over the whole body (Figure 10.6). They are at first tense but later flaccid, when they burst easily. Finger pressure causes sidewards extension of the blisters and firmly stroking the skin causes a blister (Nikolsky sign). The skin around the blister appears normal to the naked eye. The erosion left after the blister has burst is larger than the original blister and heals slowly without scar formation.

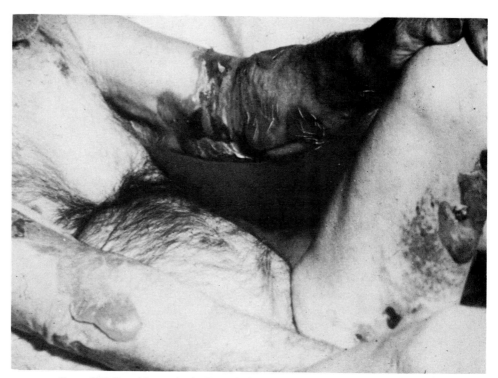

Figure 10.6. Pemphigus vulgaris. Extensive involvement of skin with thin-walled bullae.

Oral involvement is common in this disease and may precede the skin manifestations of it. Blisters similar to those on the skin appear and burst quickly to leave large erosions. They appear on the lips, cheeks, palate, floor of the mouth and on the tongue. The oral lesions are painful and distressing to the patient. Because the blisters break easily and because the erosions are particularly painful the patient may present with a complaint of 'recurring ulcers', failing to mention or notice the blisters which precede the erosions.

Smears for cytology taken from a blister or beneath the edge of an erosion are helpful in diagnosis and should be examined for acantholytic epithelial cells. These are small, rounded epithelial cells with hyperchromatic nuclei and basophilic cytoplasm which occur singly or in small clumps. The finding of such cells strongly suggests the diagnosis. They may be found in a less acantholytic form in familial benign chronic pemphigus (see above) but not in the other bullous diseases. Biopsy will reveal an intra-epithelial bulla resulting from cleavage within the epithelium just superficial to the basal cell layer. The space formed is filled with clear fluid containing acantholytic cells which, like the epithelial cells with malformed nuclei found in viral infections, are called Tzanck cells although they are quite different from these. A biopsy may be taken from the edge of an erosion or of apparently normal mucous membrane if an intact blister cannot be obtained. Finally, immunofluorescent techniques may be used to identify the intercellular substance antibodies referred to above.

Treatment of this disease is best undertaken by a dermatologist or other physician. Corticosteroids, often in high dosage, are used to break the tendency to blister formation and the patient is maintained on as small a dose as is necessary to prevent recurrence.

Pemphigus vegetans is less common than pemphigus vulgaris. Papillomatous hyperplasia of the epithelium occurs, producing 'vegetations' which become purulent and associated with inflammation. In other respects the disease resembles pemphigus vulgaris.

Bullous Pemphigoid

This is a disease of the elderly, dominated by its skin manifestations. Oral lesions may occur but only in a minority of cases. Immunofluorescent techniques have identified the presence of basement membrane antibodies in bullous pemphigoid, and the intercellular antibodies present in pemphigus vulgaris are lacking. It is suggested that antibody binding to antigen in the basement membrane occurs with the activation of complement and attracts polymorphonuclear leucocytes. Lysosomal material released from these cells as they disintegrate causes separation between epithelium and corium. Such ideas have not yet been substantiated and further knowledge is required of the precise mechanism of the production of the bullae in pemphigoid.

The bullae on the skin are often preceded by erythema and are large, tense, and frequently contain blood. They are robust and rupture late, leaving a relatively small erosion which heals with scarring. Oral lesions are less common and less dramatic than the skin manifestations.

Histology in bullous pemphigoid reveals a subepidermal bulla without acantholysis. The disease is best treated by a dermatologist who is likely to assess the patient most carefully since bullae of the type described above are one of the possible non-metastatic markers of internal malignancy.

Benign Mucous Membrane Pemphigoid

This disease bears some resemblance to bullous pemphigoid described above but differs from it in that the mucous membranes bear the brunt of involvement, the skin often escaping.

The aetiology of the disease is unknown. Antibodies to basement membrane material, as occur in bullous pemphigoid, have been discovered very recently in benign mucous membrane pemphigoid, although it must be emphasized that the immunology of the bullous diseases is by no means completely understood at the present time.

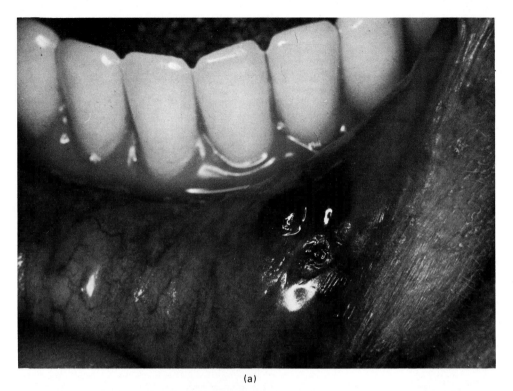

(a)

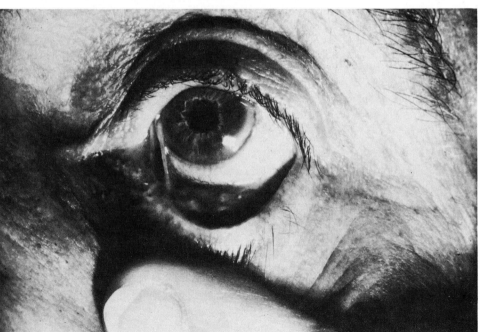

(b)

Figure 10.7. Benign mucous membrane pemphigoid: (a) blood filled bullae on labial mucosa; (b) corneal scarring.

Benign mucous membrane pemphigoid occurs more often in females than in males, with peak incidence in the fifth decade. Skin manifestations occur in a minority of cases as small tense bullae on an erythematous base and often recurring in one site. The conjunctiva and mucous membrane surfaces of the nose, larynx, pharynx, oesophagus, anus, penis, vulva and vagina may be affected. The erosions left as the bullae break heal with scarring and this is particularly hazardous in the eye and in the oesophagus. In the eye, adhesions may develop between the palpebral and the bulbar conjunctiva with loss of the palpebral fissure, eventual opacity of the cornea, and even blindness (Figure 10.7).

In the mouth, the masticatory surfaces are particularly affected and often the gingivae bear the brunt of involvement. The bullae are thick walled and may persist for a few days. They are blood-filled and tense. On breaking, they leave erosions which heal slowly, the mucous membrane becoming erythematous and fragile in appearance. The disease produces one form of desquamative gingivitis, this term being used in a descriptive sense as a non-specific manifestation of a variety of diseases. Benign mucous membrane pemphigoid and erosive lichen planus are the usual causes of this form of gingivitis, but other causes such as oestrogen imbalance have been implicated in some cases.

Benign mucous membrane pemphigoid is characterized by subepidermal blister formation and there is no acantholysis. Plasma cells and eosinophils form a non-specific chronic reaction in the underlying corium.

The disease is long-lasting and tends to persist with periods of activity alternating with inactivity for several years. Topical corticosteroid preparations may be useful during exacerbations, used with proper care, and systemic corticosteroid therapy is employed when eye or oesophageal involvement is severe.

Dermatitis Herpetiformis

This is an uncommon chronic disease of unknown aetiology but which is commonly associated with small bowel changes indistinguishable from those which occur in coeliac disease (gluten-sensitive enteropathy). The disease has a peak incidence in the fourth and fifth decades of life and more often in men than in women. A sensation of burning and itching precedes the appearance of erythematous papules and bulla. Healing is accompanied by pigmentation of the skin. Bullae may occur in the mouth and leave extensive erosions as they break. The bullae are subepithelial in position and characteristically eosinophils are prominent in them and in the underlying corium.

Remission of the disease may be produced by sulphapyridine (dapsone) and the use of this drug provides a helpful therapeutic test.

COLLAGEN DISEASES AFFECTING THE SKIN AND MUCOUS MEMBRANES

Systemic lupus erythematosus, chronic discoid lupus erythematosus and *scleroderma* are considered in Chapter 17.

FURTHER READING

Milne, J. A. (1972) *An Introduction to the Diagnostic Histopathology of the Skin.* London: Arnold.
Shafer, W. G., Hine, M. K. & Levy, B. M. (1974) Chapter 16 in *A Textbook of Oral Pathology,* 3rd ed. Philadelphia, London, Toronto: W. B. Saunders.

chapter 11

Gastroenterological Disease

OESOPHAGEAL REFLUX

Oesophageal or gastric reflux is sometimes associated with diaphragmatic hernia, and it causes burning substernal or epigastric discomfort after heavy meals, between meals or nocturnally. These symptoms are aggravated by bending or stooping, and regurgitation of bitter gastric contents into the mouth may also occur. Patients may complain of substernal pain, which can spread upwards into the neck and which may mimic the pain of cardiac origin. Such patients also complain occasionally of a burning, painful tongue but it is not clear whether this is due to acid reflux or to the iron deficiency resulting from the chronic blood loss sometimes found in this disorder. Loss of tooth structure due to acid erosion may occur (Chapter 20).

PATERSON—KELLY (PLUMMER—VINSON) SYNDROME

This syndrome of dysphagia, iron deficiency anaemia and atrophic changes in the oral mucosa is described in Chapter 6.

PEPTIC ULCERATION

In the past, a common aetiology or other link between oral aphthous ulceration and peptic ulceration has been suggested but it seems likely that the incidence of peptic ulcers in patients with oral ulceration is not excessive and that these diseases do not have a common aetiology. However, individual oral ulcer patients with dyspepsia require proper investigation and treatment of their gastric complaint and this is outside the dentist's scope. In addition, the corticosteroid preparations used in the treatment of oral aphthae should be restricted in a patient who has gastric symptoms, according to the advice of the patient's physician.

INTESTINAL MALABSORPTION

In the most common form of intestinal malabsorption, the patient is unable to tolerate the gluten present in wheat products. This disease, also called gluten enteropathy or non-tropical sprue, occurs as childhood or adult coeliac disease (Figure 11.1) and the latter may also be referred to as idiopathic steatorrhoea. Many patients with the disease have symptoms of a gastrointestinal disorder, or obvious signs of malabsorption, and these lead to the diagnosis. In other patients with the disorder, however, the signs and symptoms are so minor as to escape notice and the diagnosis is not made. Such patients may present with oral symptoms and the proper investigation of these leads to diagnosis.

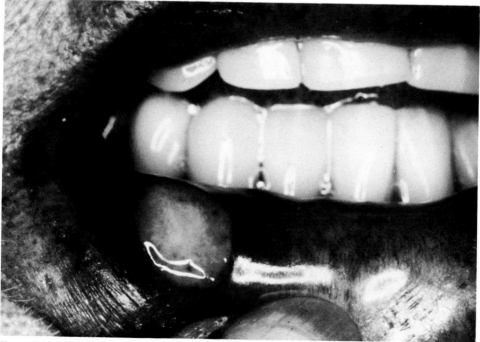

Figure 11.1 Ulceration of the lip in adult coeliac disease. Oral ulceration was the first manifestation of malabsorption in this case.

Diarrhoea is the most common complaint in gluten enteropathy but it may be absent or the patient may be constipated. Abdominal distension, excessive flatus and bouts of colicky abdominal pain also occur. Weight loss and weakness, or a failure to grow and thrive in children, result from the malabsorption which may also cause anaemia due to deficient intake of iron, vitamin B_{12} and folic acid, either separately or in combination.

Glossitis is a common finding in untreated cases and, when it is severe, the tongue is fiery red, as is the whole oral mucosa. Angular cheilitis and minor oral ulcers also occur and these are sufficient reasons for detailed questioning of all oral ulcer patients as to possible gastrointestinal symptoms, and for haematological testing which should include, in patients with a long history of recurrent oral ulceration, estimations of iron, vitamin B_{12} and folic acid levels since these may be reduced in the absence of significant anaemia. Suspicious features in the case history or on investigation call for more thorough gastroenterological investigation which should precede any attempt at treatment by excluding gluten from the diet or by replacement therapy.

It is not clear whether the oral lesions which occur in malabsorption are a manifestation of nutritional deficiency caused by the failure to absorb or another effect of the basic defect causing the malabsorption.

ULCERATIVE COLITIS

This is an inflammatory disease which affects the mucosa and submucosa of the colon and rectum, with a peak incidence in the third decade. The onset is often insidious, with mild symptoms of abdominal discomfort and malaise, but there may be a more abrupt beginning with fever. Later, there is crampy abdominal pain, rectal bleeding and diarrhoea with tenesmus; the stools containing blood, pus and mucus. The disease is characterized by periods of remission and exacerbation.

Skin lesions such as erythema nodosum and papulonecrotic lesions occur in a small proportion of patients with ulcerative colitis and are thought to be associated with underlying autoimmune mechanisms. Specific oral lesions are uncommon, although pyostomatitis may occur as necrotic grey patches, sometimes ramifying to produce a complex pattern and eventually giving a red papilliferous appearance called pyostomatitis vegetans. The oral lesions may or may not wax and wane with the activity of the colitis but investigation and treatment by a physician are required. Oral ulcers identical to aphthae also appear in this disorder.

CROHN'S DISEASE (REGIONAL ENTERITIS)

This is a chronic inflammatory disease, chiefly affecting the terminal ileum and causing narrowing of it. The patient experiences recurrent episodes of crampy abdominal pain accompanied by fever and diarrhoea. Malnutrition and anaemia result, and specific deficiencies of protein, calcium, vitamin D and vitamin B_{12}, etc. produce a wide variety of ill effects. Perianal abscesses may occur as part of the primary disease process.

Oral ulceration is a presenting symptom in about 1 per cent of cases of Crohn's disease and may predate other symptoms. The oral lesions may occur on the gums, buccal mucosa or lips (Figure 11.2). The gingival lesions appear as longstanding, purplish-red, tender or non-tender, non-haemorrhagic enlargements occurring in areas

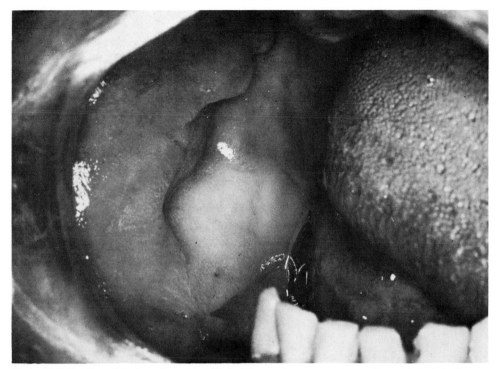

Figure 11.2. Swelling of the buccal mucosa with 'cobblestone' appearance in a patient with Crohn's disease.

of good plaque control. Ulcers, often linear and persisting for several months or years, have been described on the lips or buccal sulcus. Buccal mucosal lesions have included formations of granulation tissue, a general redness, or a thickening with folding and ridging. Elongated, denture granuloma-like masses in dentulous mouths, sometimes described as indurated and sometimes bilateral, have also been described on the buccal mucosa or in the buccal sulci. Some patients have had swollen lips due either to involvement of the lip itself or to chronic lymphatic obstruction as a consequence of intra-oral disease (Figure 11.3). Persistence and resistance to treatment are characteristic of the oral lesions, the severity of which appears to mirror the severity of the disease elsewhere rather than the deficiency of iron, B_{12} or folate.

Biopsy of the oral lesions is often helpful in diagnosis and occasionally reveals the non-caseating granulomas, with epithelioid cells, giant cells and peripheral lymphocytes, which occur in Crohn's disease; but more frequently focal collections of lymphocytes and other non-specific signs of chronic inflammation are found.

INTESTINAL POLYPOSIS

Intestinal polyps may occur singly or in a multiple form. It is usual to refer to the latter form as polyposis. A number of varieties of polyposis exist and two of these have relevance in respect of oral disease, namely Peutz—Jeghers syndrome and Gardner's syndrome.

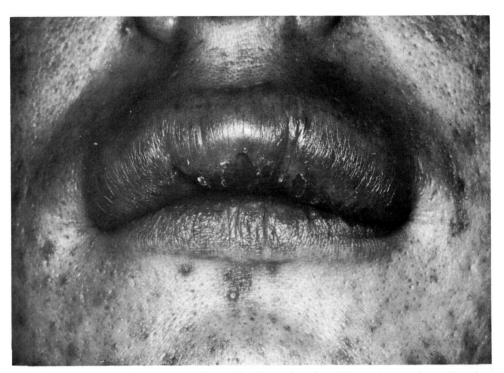

Figure 11.3. Uniform swelling of the upper lip with fissuring and erosions. This can be an early manifestation of Crohn's disease.

The Peutz—Jeghers syndrome consists of mucocutaneous pigmentation and gastrointestinal polyposis and is an inherited disease. The pigmentation is arranged in oval, round or irregular brown or black macules which first appear in early childhood. In the mouth the buccal mucosa and lips (Figure 11.4) are most often affected but the pigmented macules may also be found on the palate, gingiva and, although rarely, on the tongue. Similar pigmentation may occur in the nasal mucosa, conjunctiva and rectal mucosa. The cutaneous pigmentation occurs around the mouth, nostrils and eyes and on the hands, feet and trunk, and is caused by the presence of melanin-containing cells in the basal layer of the epithelium and by collections of melanophores in the corium. This pigmentation differs from freckles in that it occurs in subjects of all complexions, including negroes; it is darker, and the macules are more discrete; it is chiefly arranged around the mouth, nose or eyes rather than the bridge of the nose and cheeks; it occurs intra-orally; and it develops in infancy or early childhood. The mucosal pigmentation does not disappear with age, but the skin spots fade in adult life. The polyposis is chiefly in the small intestine, although the large bowel is affected in about 50 per cent of cases. The polyps are usually few in number and may cause obstruction or bleeding. They are formed by tree-like malformations of the muscularis mucosae and the epithelial covering is essentially normal, the whole lesion being classified as a hamartoma (malformation) rather than as an adenoma. The polyposis is not considered to be premalignant, although genuine examples of intestinal malignancy in the syndrome have been reported and doubt exists as to whether it is completely innocent. Polyps may occur in the urinary tract, and in the nose as well as in the mouth.

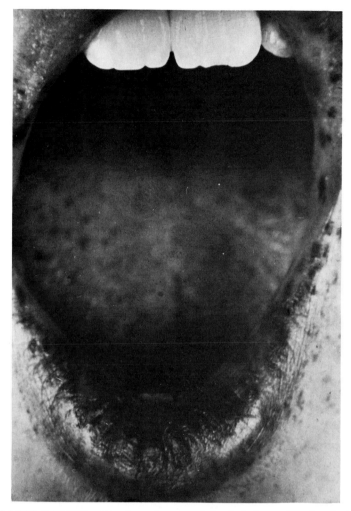

Figure 11.4. Labial pigmentation occurring as brown spots in a typical case of Peutz — Jeghers syndrome.

Gardner's syndrome consists of soft- and hard-tissue tumours in association with colonic polyposis. The syndrome is inherited and when one parent is affected 50 per cent of offspring will be similarly affected. The soft-tissue lesions consist of sebaceous cysts, subcutaneous fibromas and other masses of fibrous tissue. The hard-tissue swellings usually occur in association with skull and facial bones and appear as osteomas, the ramus of the mandible and sinuses being likely sites. Intestinal polyposis may occur as early as the second decade and malignant change is likely unless prophylactic surgical excision of the affected part of the bowel is undertaken. The innocent soft-tissue swellings may predate the signs of intestinal polyposis by many years and if diagnosis is delayed until intestinal symptoms appear, about 40 per cent of patients develop malignancy. Thus, it is vital that the dentist be aware of the condition since he may be able to suggest the diagnosis at a stage when prophylactic surgery will prevent the serious complications of the disease.

HEPATITIS AND CIRRHOSIS

The major sign of liver disease is jaundice or icterus, a yellowish discoloration of the plasma, skin and mucous membrane due to staining by bile pigment and usually detectable when the serum bilirubin is in excess of 34 μmol/l (2 mg/100 cc). Jaundice is best seen in the conjunctivae, but is also apparent in the labial mucous membrane, when the lips are compressed with a glass slide, and in the palate.

Glossitis or atrophy of the tongue occurs in about half the patients with portal cirrhosis, perhaps due to concomitant vitamin B_{12} deficiency. Gingival bleeding is found as part of a generalized bleeding tendency in some patients with liver damage, as in post-necrotic cirrhosis. In addition, patients with liver failure may exhibit 'foetor hepaticus', a peculiar sweet or amine malodour of the breath.

Asymptomatic enlargement of the parotid glands (see page 165) may occur in chronic alcoholics with hepatic cirrhosis. Normally, the parotid is not palpable and a concavity exists between the superior ramus of the mandible and the sternomastoid muscle. In chronic alcoholics the enlarged parotid gland is palpable and fills the concavity referred to. The swelling is firm and rubbery and usually bilateral and symmetrical. Infrequently, such patients have concomitant enlargement of the sub-maxillary salivary gland, termed 'sialosis'.

A positive association between cancer of the mouth and pharynx, and liver cirrhosis, heavy alcohol consumption and heavy smoking has been detected. It would appear that an association exists for each of the factors separately but the precise relationship between liver cirrhosis and oral cancer is not understood at present.

MUCOVISCIDOSIS (FIBROCYSTIC DISEASE OF THE PANCREAS)

Fibrocystic disease of the pancreas is an inherited disease which affects mucus-secreting and non-mucus-secreting exocrine glands. The chief effects occur in the bronchi and lungs where bronchial obstruction and secondary infection lead to bronchiectasis. The salivary glands are also involved in the process. The submaxillary salivary glands enlarge and there is a reduction in their output. The parotid glands are less affected. Few dental studies exist but there is said to be an exaggerated tendency to calculus formation in children who have the disease. However, the caries incidence is not excessive. Changes in salivary secretion may occur (see page 145).

Grey-black or brown tooth discoloration has been described in mucoviscidosis but it is probable that the discoloration is due to the tetracycline therapy these patients so often receive to control chest infection.

part 3

DISEASE OF SALIVARY GLANDS

chapter 12

Disorders of Salivary Gland Function and Composition

Those factors and disease states which alter the rate of flow and composition of saliva are described in this chapter. As an introduction, however, a brief description of the development, structure and function of the salivary glands is presented.

DEVELOPMENT, STRUCTURE AND FUNCTION

Development

The salivary glands develop from proliferating buds of oral epithelium. Invasion of the underlying mesenchyma is followed by budding of the gland primordia. After budding, the terminal portions branch and form ducts which end as bulbous terminals from which the acinar element develops.

The earliest changes are noted in about the fourth week of intra-uterine life in the parotid gland, followed by submandibular, sublingual and minor glands at 6, 8 and 12 weeks, respectively. The glands become invested in connective tissue, the parotid gland being the last of the major glands to become encapsulated. As a consequence lymphoid tissue may become entrapped within the gland. Sebaceous elements may also be present and, together with lymphoid tissue, may become the seat of pathological change in later life. Functional activity of the glands does not occur during fetal life.

Structure

Fundamentally, the salivary glands comprise acinar cells and a duct system which is both intra- and extraglandular, divided into lobules by connective tissue which supports the neurovascular elements. The mechanism of secretion is complex but is regulated by the autonomic nervous system.

Histologically, acinar cells may be mucous or serous. Duct cells vary in size, shape and staining quality but intercalated, striated and excretory duct types are recognized. Myoepithelial cells are elongated and lie between the base of the acinar or intercalated duct cells and the basement membrane. They have structural and functional similarity to smooth muscle cells. A further cell type is the oncocyte, a larger, eosinophilic and granular cell. Its function is obscure but hyperlasia of this cell is noted as a part of the ageing process.

Function

The function of the salivary glands is to produce saliva which physically keeps the oral cavity moist, facilitates speech and lubricates food for chewing and swallowing. Saliva is essential for taste acuity and oral hygiene. The secretion of saliva is subject to many variables, including time of day, age, sex and gland involved. The composition of saliva, too, is variable and many constituents are flow-rate dependent. Saliva has important protective and antibacterial functions. Largely by virtue of the local production of immunoglobulin — IgA with small amounts of IgG and IgM — the salivary glands may influence the course of oral and dental disease.

FUNCTIONAL DISORDERS

The quantitative production of saliva has been the subject of many studies and the conflicting results may be due to the variations in methods used and in the experimental conditions. The secretion of saliva is affected also by a number of psychological and environmental factors, making the establishment of exact normal values difficult.

Factors Influencing Salivary Flow Rate

In addition to organic disease of the salivary glands, mechanical stimulation, age, sex-distribution factors and diet may lead to alterations in the rate of salivary flow. Dehydration of the body causes a diminution, and hyperhydration an increase, in salivary secretion. Mental stress, anxiety and psychopathological emotional states, fatigue, infection and room temperature may all lead to a diminution of salivary gland flow rate. The effects of drugs, especially some tranquillizers and ganglion-blocking agents, have been shown to cause marked oral dryness. Diurnal variation of salivary flow must also be taken into consideration and, therefore, the time of collection as well as the method of collection are important factors which influence the secretion of saliva. Recently, light deprivation has been shown to decrease salivary flow.

XEROSTOMIA

Xerostomia may be a sign or a symptom. It is a fairly common clinical complaint which can in some cases be extremely distressing to the patient. Although xerostomia is a primary complaint in one in 1500 patients attending the Glasgow Dental Hospital, it is interesting to note that, on enquiry, one in ten patients had experienced dryness of the mouth as a regular symptom. It is useful to distinguish between true or primary xerostomia, where a pathological lesion is present in the salivary glands as a manifestation of either localized or generalized disease, and symptomatic or secondary xerostomia, where no salivary lesion is present. The effects upon the oral mucosa include epithelial atrophy, inflammation, fissuring and ulceration (Figure 12.1). In addition to xerostomia, the patient may complain of a burning sensation, sore tongue, oral soreness and ulceration and difficulty with denture retention. Xerostomia, of whatever cause, predisposes to infection of the pharynx and salivary glands and to a marked increase in dental caries.

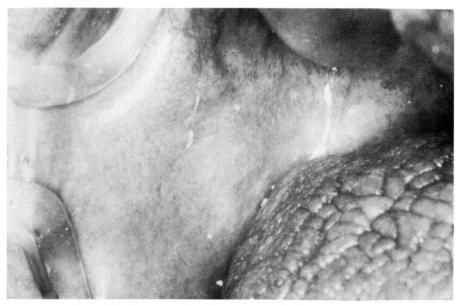

Figure 12.1. Profound oral dryness in a patient with Sjögren's syndrome.

The causes of xerostomia are numerous. As described earlier in this chapter, emotional and anxiety states and the effect of various drugs such as tranquillizers, hypotensive agents and medications containing atropine are implicated in symptomatic xerostomia. Other factors include pernicious anaemia, iron deficiency anaemia, loss of fluid through haemorrhage, sweating, diarrhoea or vomiting, the polyuria of diabetes mellitus and diabetes insipidus and various vitamin and hormonal deficiencies. Primary xerostomia may be due to absence of salivary tissue, irradiation, glandular infection or obstruction and systemic disease such as Sjögren's syndrome in which the salivary glands are involved. Disease affecting either the afferent or efferent portion of the neural transmission reflex will affect flow. When the causes of xerostomia are studied, a striking feature is the high percentage of patients in whom systemic factors are implicated.

Treatment is aimed at seeking and removing the cause. The use of a glycerine-and-lemon mouthwash is helpful in alleviating the symptoms in most cases. The stimulation of salivary flow by pilocarpine has been used by some workers. The use of solutions containing sodium chloride and sodium bicarbonate may also be of value as mouthwashes. Recently, synthetic saliva, containing carboxymethylcellulose, sorbitol and optimal quantities of salts, has been developed and appears promising. In the general management of xerostomia, strict attention to oral hygiene is essential and microbiological examination at regular intervals is of value if recurrent oral infection is to be avoided.

SIALORRHOEA

Increased salivation (sialorrhoea or ptyalism) is relatively uncommon. The predisposing factors include acute inflammatory conditions leading to stomatitis, such as herpetic and aphthous ulceration. Increased salivation is commonly encountered during the period when teeth are erupting in young individuals. Patients with neurological disturbances such as mental retardation, parkinsonism, schizophrenia and epilepsy (Figure 12.2) are subject to sialorrhoea. Drooling or pooling of saliva in the mouth in these cases may be due to loss of muscle control or other factors rather than to increased flow rate per se. The rate of salivary flow may be increased in mercury poisoning, acrodynia and rabies. In familial dysautonomia, a syndrome thought to result from an inborn error in catecholamine metabolism, increased salivation, especially during excitement, is a frequent finding.

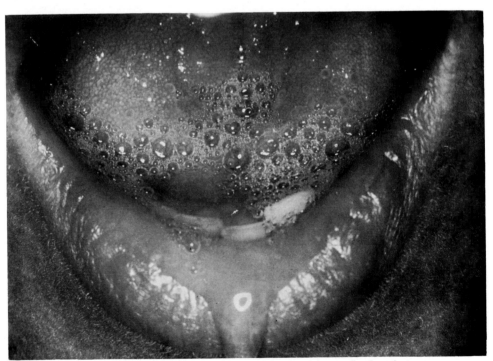

Figure 12.2. Pooling of saliva in the floor of the mouth in an epileptic patient.

With regard to treatment, attention to the cause together with the use of bicarbonate mouthwashes are helpful for this distressing condition. The use of anti-cholinergic drugs which have an atropine-like or nerve-sectioning effect may be necessary in severe cases.

CHANGES IN SALIVARY COMPOSITION

Alterations of salivary composition have been reported in various disease states affecting salivary glands or other body tissues. With the advent of better methods for the collection of saliva and the availability of new analytical techniques there has been an increase in biochemical measurements of salivary constituents. Many of the changes in biochemical composition found merely reflect changes in blood, plasma or serum levels, and while they may be of research interest are not of diagnostic significance. The use of saliva might be advantageous when frequent monitoring of a constituent such as electrolytes or urea is required, thus avoiding repeated venepuncture. There are instances where changes in salivary composition have proved helpful in clinical assessment and diagnosis of patients.

Problems in Interpreting Studies of Salivary Constituents

When interpreting the significance of the concentration of a salivary constituent it is necessary to consider some of the factors which might influence the interpretation.
The influence of the following factors should be considered:

1. Species
2. Sex
3. Source of saliva
4. Nature of stimulus
5. Duration of the stimulus
6. Rest transients
7. Flow rate
8. Plasma level
9. Diet
10. Hormones
11. Diurnal variation
12. Drugs

All or any one of these factors may affect the level of a particular salivary constituent. It is essential, therefore, to define the conditions under which a sample of saliva is obtained before any significance can be attributed to the results of its biochemical analysis.

Diseases in which Alterations in Salivary Composition Occur

These diseases include fibrocystic disease, thyroid disease, sialosis, hypertension, diabetes and connective tissue diseases, and they will now be discussed. It should be noted that the value of these findings to clinical practice awaits further study. At the present time their usefulness is largely limited to research.

Fibrocystic Disease

The exocrine glands, in particular the pancreas, salivary, sweat and bronchial glands, are affected in this condition. Marked changes occur in salivary composition. In parotid saliva, there are elevated concentrations of sodium, calcium and phosphorus and high levels of urea and uric acid have also been reported. In the submandibular saliva, elevated protein, glycoproteins, calcium, phosphorus, sodium, chloride, urea and uric acid are noted. (See also Chapter 11.)

Thyroid Disease

The thyroid and salivary glands share a similar iodide-concentrating mechanism. In the thyroid, inorganic iodide is taken up from the plasma and is concentrated in the thyroid to many times the plasma level. It is then conjugated with protein and by a series of steps is transformed to the thyroid hormones tri-iodothyronine (T_3) and thyroxine (T_4) which are secreted. Similarly, in the salivary glands the iodide is concentrated from the plasma but conjugation with protein does not occur, the inorganic iodide being secreted in the saliva. Measurement of the plasma inorganic iodide (PII) is of value in assessing thyroid disease such as non-toxic goitre and in studying the action of anti-thyroid drugs. The plasma/iodide ratio, normally at least 10, has value in studies of the iodide trapping mechanism.

Sialosis

In this condition there is painless bilateral enlargement of the parotid glands (see Chapter 14). An increase in the parotid and submandibular potassium levels may be observed and may have diagnostic value.

Other Systemic Diseases

As well as fibrocystic disease, abnormal salivary protein patterns have been associated with various pathological conditions. These include diabetes mellitus, hypertension and osteoporosis, connective tissue disorders and sarcoidosis.

THE SECRETION OF DRUGS IN SALIVA

The salivary glands are usually described as having an excretory function because of their handling and secretion of certain substances such as iodide, thiocyanate, mercury and lead. Of course, if such a substance (e.g. iodide) is then swallowed and reabsorbed it cannot really be regarded as having been excreted from the body. Drugs, or substances derived from them, may be secreted in saliva; for example, cough mixtures contain large amounts of iodide which, after ingestion, is secreted in saliva. Alkaloids such as morphine, metronidazole, a drug used in the treatment of acute ulcerative gingivitis, and ethyl alcohol have all been detected under their systemic administration.

FURTHER READING

Jenkins, G. N. (1978) *The Physiology of the Mouth,* 3rd ed. Oxford: Blackwell Scientific.
Mason, D. K. & Chisholm, D. M. (1975) *Salivary Glands in Health and Disease.* London, Philadelphia, Toronto: W. B. Saunders.

chapter 13

Infection, Obstruction and Trauma

Infection
Obstruction and Trauma

INFECTION

Inflammatory disorders of the major salivary glands which result from bacterial or viral infection are the most common salivary gland diseases. On rare occasions an allergic reaction may result in a sialadenitis. Infection of the salivary glands is manifested by painful swelling of the affected gland with an alteration in salivary secretion rate and character.

Acute Sialadenitis of Bacterial Origin

Predisposing factors include reduction of salivary flow which may be a postoperative complication, especially of abdominal surgery when the patient is debilitated or dehydrated. Acute parotitis may follow the use of drugs such as phenothiazine and its derivatives which cause xerostomia and thus predispose to ascending infections. The condition may also represent an acute exacerbation of a low-grade chronic non-specific sialadenitis. Clinically, acute sialadenitis is a painful swelling (Figure 13.1). A purulent discharge (Figure 13.2) may be expressed from the duct orifice by digital pressure over the affected gland.

It is to be noted that the introduction of sulphonamides and antibiotics led to a marked reduction in the incidence of acute parotitis. With the emergence of antibiotic-resistant strains of *Staphylococcus aureus*, however, acute parotitis has become more prevalent again.

Chronic Sialadenitis of Bacterial Origin

As a complication of duct obstruction chronic sialadenitis is not uncommon, especially in the submandibular gland. In general, the aetiological factors are similar to those for acute sialadenitis. The condition is usually unilateral, with pain and swelling in the pre-auricular, retromandibular or submandibular region. On occasions, there may be difficulty in distinguishing submandibular sialadenitis from sublingual or subman-dibular cellulitis due to other causes. However, the affected duct orifice is reddened and a purulent, rather salty-tasting discharge from the duct of the affected gland may be present.

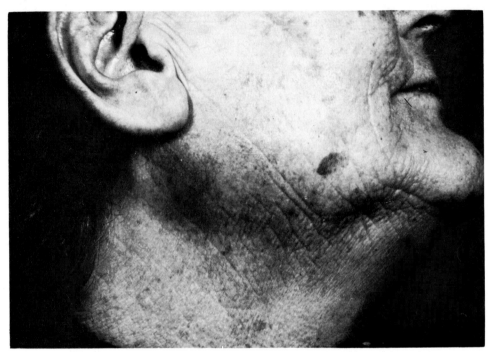

Figure 13.1. Acute sialadenitis of the parotid gland.

Recurrent parotitis is a well-documented condition and occurs in both adults and children. The attacks of parotitis consist of sudden pain and swelling, usually lasting for a period of three to seven days, in the region of one or both parotid glands. The affected gland may remain slightly enlarged between the attacks which vary from one every few weeks to once or twice a year. Fortunately, there is a marked tendency of the condition to resolve completely in children once puberty is attained. Those patients whose sialograms show little or no duct dilation and whose flow rates are within normal limits are more likely to recover spontaneously.

In the management of sialadenitis, culture of saliva, collected by catheterizing the duct, or of pus from the duct should be carried out so that appropriate antibiotic therapy may be instigated. Sialography should be performed to differentiate between those cases with and those without main duct change. Stimulation of flow by chewing or massage prevents stagnation. In view of the frequent spontaneous recovery after puberty, surgical intervention should be avoided in cases of recurrent sialadenitis of childhood.

The salivary glands are seldom involved in specific inflammatory disorders. On rare occasions, however, they may be the site of granulomatous disorders, such as tuberculosis, syphilis and sarcoidosis, and are affected as part of these systemic disease processes.

Mikulicz's syndrome is often applied to the condition of bilateral enlargement of the salivary and lacrimal glands due to a known cause such as specific granulomas or lymphoid neoplasia. Actinomycosis of the parotid gland has been reported but is exceedingly rare. Resolution is usually achieved by appropriate treatment of the systemic disorder.

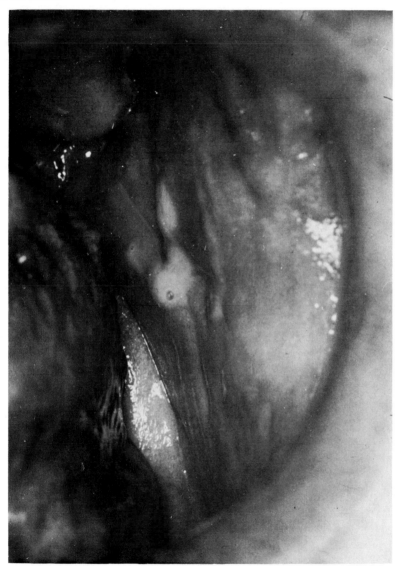

Figure 13.2. Purulent discharge from the duct orifice of the L parotid gland.

Viral Sialadenitis

Mumps is an acute, infectious, viral disease that primarily affects the salivary glands, especially the parotids (Figure 13.3). It occurs in all areas of the world and is the most common of all salivary gland diseases. It is an endemic disease throughout the year in temperate climates but usually increases seasonally, in late winter and spring. Mumps virus, which has an incubation period of two to three weeks, is transmitted by direct contact or in droplets of saliva. The disease affects both sexes equally, and is usually contracted by children and young adults. The onset is sudden, with fever, headache and painful swelling. Classically, only one gland is affected at first. The swelling reaches a maximum within two days and diminishes over an additional week.

Adults who contract the disease may develop serious complications, such as orchitis and oöphoritis, although sterility is rare. Other organs which may be affected are the pancreas, liver, kidney and nervous system.

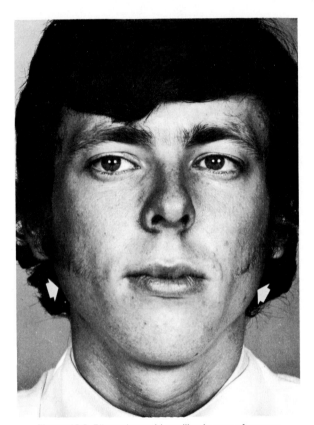

Figure 13.3. Bilateral parotid swelling in case of mumps.

A durable immunity results from mumps and in adults is detected by their reacting to skin-test antigen and by the presence of complement-fixing antibodies. In serum, a rise in antibody titre, detected by complement fixation, occurs within one week. The virus may be detected by complement fixation in saliva two to three days before the onset of sialadenitis and for about six days afterwards. Treatment is usually symptomatic — bed rest, analgesics and a fluid diet — with isolation for six to ten days.

It is important to note that parotitis may be caused by other viruses, such as coxsackie virus type A, echovirus, choriomeningitis virus and para-influenza types 1 and 2 viruses.

Salivary Gland Inclusion Disease

This rare condition usually affects infants in the first few days of life. Infection occurs transplacentally. Adults are rarely affected, but in the known cases there is an association with severe debilitating diseases such as leukaemia or a terminal neoplasm.

Inflammation of the minor salivary glands may occur as part of a local disease process or may reflect a generalized systemic disease.

Cheilitis glandularis apostematosa, in which the lips, especially the lower, become swollen, is a rare condition. The cause is unknown. The condition is painless and appears to affect males more than females. A thick viscid mucus can be expressed from the glands in the affected region. Although a labial sialadenitis is present, the underlying pathogenetic mechanism appears to be one of acinar and duct hypertrophy.

Allergic Sialadenitis

Salivary gland enlargement as a localized allergic reaction is rare. Among the allergens reported are various foods, drugs such as chloramphenicol and oxytetracycline, various pollens and heavy metals.

It has been suggested that eosinophils in saliva and blood eosinophil count may be helpful diagnostically. In the treatment of allergic sialadenitis, antihistamines are of limited value. Clearly, the offending allergen should be avoided.

OBSTRUCTION AND TRAUMA

Obstruction to the flow of saliva may follow lesions of the duct papilla, the presence of a salivary calculus (or sialolith) and pressure from lesions within and outside the duct wall. Salivary fistula formation and Frey's syndrome may be complications of trauma to the parotid region. Mucoceles are common lesions and both traumatic and obstructive factors have been implicated in their formation.

The commonest cause of papillary obstruction is trauma from, for example, a sharp cusp of a tooth, faulty restorations, projecting clasps, over-extended denture flanges and dentures with high occlusal planes. Alternatively, a soft-tissue lesion such as an ulcer may lead to acute papillary obstruction.

Sialolithiasis

Calcification leading to obstruction within duct lumens can be found in many organs of the human body, most often in the urinary tract, gall-bladder and submandibular salivary gland (Figure 13.4). They may also occur, however, in the parotid, sublingual and minor salivary glands, and the pancreas. It is of interest that, although the parotid gland is most commonly affected by adenitis, sialolithiasis is less common.

Adults are more commonly affected, although sialolithiasis may occur in children, and the classical clinical signs and symptoms are those of pain and sudden enlargement of the affected gland, especially at mealtimes. Clinical diagnosis may be confirmed visually by palpation and radiography (Figure 13.5). Treatment, depending on the site and the clinical features, is by surgical removal of the calculus — incision of the duct or dilatation of the duct orifice — although, in some cases, removal of the gland may be necessary if infection or re-infection occurs.

Salivary duct obstruction may result from stricture, especially following ulceration around a submandibular sialolith. Stricture may follow other traumatic injuries to the duct. These lesions are best treated by dilatation of the stricture with graduated sizes of lacrimal duct probes, coated with lignocaine gel. Salivary ducts may be obstructed by pressure of tumours from without. Benign neoplasms simply compress the duct although malignant lesions may also infiltrate the duct wall.

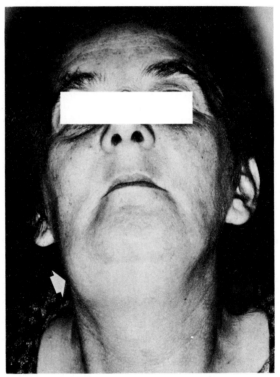

Figure 13.4. Swelling of the right submandibular gland due to the presence of a duct sialolith.

Fistula

A salivary duct fistula is defined as an abnormal communication between the duct system and the oral cavity or the skin which allows secretion of saliva externally. Although it is uncommon, external salivary duct fistula formation presents a troublesome and distressing condition for the patient. Since internal fistulae drain into the oral cavity they are asymptomatic and therefore of little consequence. A salivary duct fistula may be congenital, although more commonly it follows trauma — for example, deep laceration of the cheek, or as a complication of major gland surgery or as a result of ulceration and infection associated with sialadenitis, large calculi or tumours.

Treatment and management is primarily by surgical repair.

Frey's Syndrome

In this unusual condition, sweating and flushing of the skin over the distribution of the auriculotemporal nerve take place following a stimulus to salivary secretion. The syndrome may be a consequence of parotid surgery, temporomandibular surgery or injuries and infections in this region. The condition is thought to arise following damage to the auriculotemporal nerve which contains post-ganglionic parasympathetic fibres from the otic ganglion. These damaged fibres then become united to sympathetic nerves from the superior cervical ganglion which supplies the sweat glands of the skin.

There is no satisfactory approach to treatment.

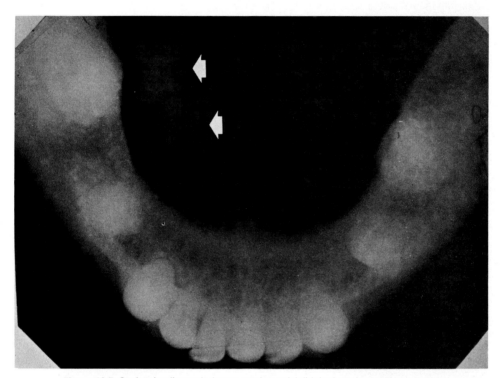

Figure 13.5. Occlusal radiograph demonstrating a sialolith in the submandibular duct.

Mucoceles

Mucoceles may be superficial or deep and may vary in size from a few millimetres to 1 cm in diameter. Those which are superficial have a bluish, translucent colour and rupture easily. Deeper-seated mucoceles have the same colour as the surrounding oral mucosa. Recurrence is common, especially of the superficial type of lesion.

Mucoceles occur most commonly in the lower lip (Figure 13.6), with a less common occurrence in the buccal mucosa and floor of mouth. The palate and upper lip are rarely involved.

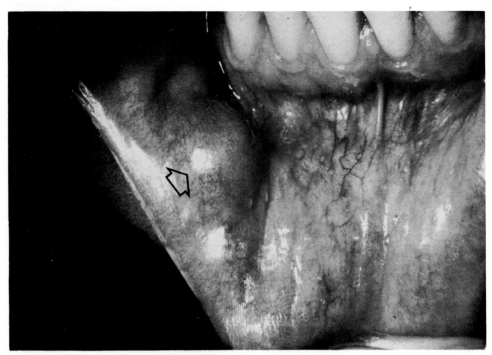

Figure 13.6. Mucocele of the lower lip.

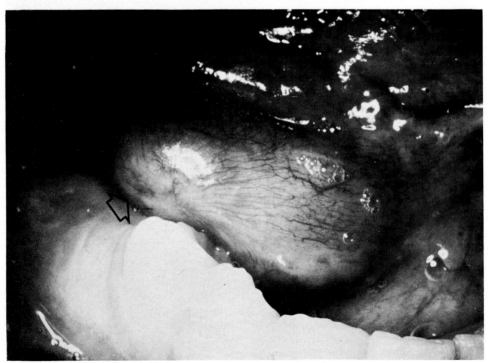

Figure 13.7. Ranula associated with the sublingual salivary gland.

Histologically, mucoceles may be graded as a mucus-extravasation cyst or a mucus-retention cyst.

The mucus-extravasation cyst is thought to be caused by mechanical trauma of minor excretory ducts leading to severance of the duct, with resultant spillage of mucus into the connective tissue stroma. The mucous pool is localized or walled off by a condensation of connective and granulation tissue. A mucus-retention cyst refers to a mucocele which results from a partial obstruction to the flow of saliva. As a consequence, the duct dilates, with a resulting cystic lesion lined by simple columnar or pseudostratified squamous epithelium.

'Ranula' is the name given to a form of mucocele which occurs in the floor of the mouth (Figure 13.7) and is associated with the ducts of the submandibular and the sublingual salivary glands. They are usually unilateral swellings, 2 to 3 cm in diameter, and are soft and fluctuant with a bluish-violet colour. Although generally painless they may interfere with speech, mastication and swallowing.

These lesions should be removed by surgical excision.

FURTHER READING

Mason, D. K. & Chisholm, D. M. (1975) *Salivary Glands in Health and Disease.* London, Philadelphia, Toronto: W. B. Saunders.

chapter 14

Tumours and Associated Conditions

Neoplasms
Sjögren's Syndrome
Lymphoepithelial Lesion
Sialosis

NEOPLASMS

Introduction

Neoplasms of the salivary glands present problems both to clinicians and pathologists, especially with regard to diagnosis, classification and nomenclature. The histological pattern and behavioural characteristics of salivary neoplasms vary considerably and it is not surprising that classifications and nomenclature based upon these criteria have led to the introduction of a confusing variety of names. It is hoped that the 1972 publication by the World Health Organization of a classification and nomenclature of salivary gland neoplasms, based upon histological type, will encourage uniformity of usage in these respects. At an international level, the comparison of incidence and response to treatment should provide important data with regard to salivary neoplasms.

The parotid glands are the most commonly affected, followed by the submandibular glands, the minor glands as a group and, finally, the sublingual glands. For the intra-oral minor glands, the palate is the commonest site of involvement. Where major studies have been undertaken there appears to be little variation with regard to incidence of salivary neoplasms in the United States, the United Kingdom and northern Europe. However, there is evidence to suggest that departure from this general view, especially in terms of tumour type and location, may occur as an expression of ethnic grouping. Thus, amongst the Chinese in Malaya, submandibular salivary neoplasms are relatively high, whilst Eskimoes appear to have a predisposition to salivary carcinoma.

It is worth noting that with regard to tumour type and location, the pleomorphic adenoma is the commonest salivary neoplasm at all locations, the adenolymphoma occurs almost exclusively in the parotid gland, and the adenoid cystic carcinoma is relatively more common in the minor than in the major glands.

Clinical Features

The majority of salivary gland neoplasms present clinically as a slowly enlarging, painless swelling. On palpation the lesions are usually firm, mobile and smooth-surfaced (Figures 14.1 and 14.2). Intra-oral lesions may become ulcerated due to masticatory trauma. In the parotid gland, the lower pole of the superficial portion of the gland is the commonest site. Those clinical features which suggest the presence of a malignant neoplasm are rapidity of growth, fixation to skin or underlying structures, pain, ulceration and motor nerve involvement. On rare occasions a salivary gland neoplasm may present at an ectopic site, such as within mandibular bone, whilst it is worth noting that the adenolymphoma may occur bilaterally in approximately 10 per cent of cases. All lesions in which neoplasia is suspected should be biopsied, care being taken to avoid 'seeding' of the tumour into the biopsy wound.

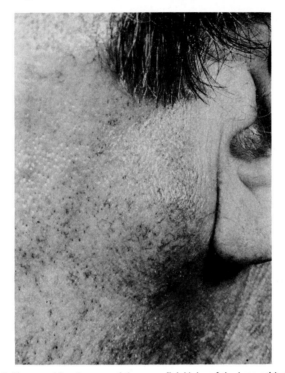

Figure 14.1. Pleomorphic adenoma of the superficial lobe of the L parotid gland.

Classification

The majority of salivary gland neoplasms fall into the recent classification laid down by the World Health Organization. As can be observed in Table 14.1 tumours may be grouped broadly into four categories as follows:

1. Epithelial tumours
2. Non-epithelial tumours
3. Unclassified tumours
4. Allied conditions

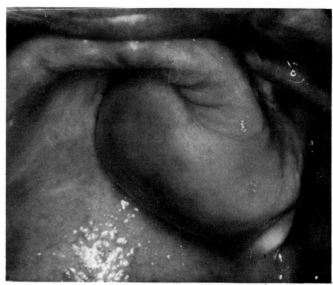

Figure 14.2. Firm swelling of palate and L tuberosity region. Histopathological examination showed a pleomorphic adenoma.

The non-epithelial tumours comprise a miscellaneous group which includes those arising from connective tissue, for example haemangioma and neurofibroma. The unclassified group can be either benign or malignant primary growths, where the histological features are such that they cannot readily be placed into either of the other two neoplastic categories. The final group of allied conditions includes the essentially

Table 14.1. *Histological typing of salivary gland tumours.*

1. Epithelial tumours

    (a) Adenomas
        (i) Pleomorphic adenoma (mixed tumour)
        (ii) Monomorphic adenomas: Adenolymphoma
                                  Oxyphilic adenoma
                                  Other types

    (b) Muco-epidermoid tumour

    (c) Acinic-cell tumour

    (d) Carcinomas
        (i)   Adenoid cystic carcinoma
        (ii) Adenocarcinoma
        (iii) Epidermoid carcinoma
        (iv) Undifferentiated carcinoma
        (v) Carcinoma in pleomorphic adenoma (malignant mixed tumour)

2. Non-epithelial tumours

3. Unclassified tumours

4. Allied conditions

    (a) Benign lymphoepithelial lesion

    (b) Sialosis

    (c) Oncocytosis

From Thackray (1972).

non-neoplastic gland enlargements such as lymphoepithelial lesion, sialosis and oncocytosis. This group is dealt with in more detail elsewhere in this text. Although the histopathological details of all these lesions are to be found in specialist tests, it seems relevant to describe briefly the main features of the epithelial tumours which may affect the salivary glands, since they are the most common.

Pathology

The histopathological features of the adenomas, muco-epidermoid tumour, acinic-cell tumour and carcinomas of salivary glands are now considered.

Pleomorphic Adenoma

This neoplasm derives its name from its 'pleomorphic' or 'mixed' cellular appearance, which indicates the appearance of the lesion histologically rather than implying a particular histogenesis. Pleomorphic adenomas of the major salivary gland range from two to five centimetres in diameter. They present macroscopically as round or ovoid, encapsulated and, on occasion, multilobular. The capsule or peripheral condensation of connective tissue varies in thickness and texture, and parts of the tumour mass may protrude through it. The tumour is usually solid, although cystic and/or haemorrhagic areas may be present. The texture of the tumour shows much variation, the variation depending largely upon the ratio of epithelial to connective tissue elements. Thus, all degrees of variation may be observed, from hard, firm, elastic or calcified tumours to soft, mucoid and cystic tumours.

By definition, the pleomorphic adenoma has a varied histological appearance. Essentially, epithelial duct cells proliferate to form sheets, cords and/or clumps of cells, many forming duct-like structures, amid a varying supporting stroma. Stromal variation, often within the one tumour, includes mucoid, myxoid, chondroid, hyaline, elastic and, occasionally, osseous change.

Monomorphic Adenomas

The monomorphic adenomas are thought to arise from duct cells which form tumours having a characteristic regular, usually glandular, pattern with no evidence of mucoid or other connective tissue stromal change. There are several varieties of monomorphic adenoma, and these are described briefly, as follows:

Oxyphilic adenoma. This tumour is characterized by the presence of large numbers of oncocytes and little supporting stroma.

Adenolymphoma. This tumour tends to be multifocal in origin. It consists of lymphoid tissue supporting epithelial cells which form double-layered structures thrown into papillary folds with large cyst-like spaces within the tumour.

Other types. These adenomas may be classified according to their morphological appearance. Thus, basal cell, tubular, trabecular (with or without cystic or papillary formations), clear-cell and alveolar adenomas have all been described. The fundamental features of all these lesions, however, is their uniformity of cell structure and absence of stromal change, which set them apart from other salivary neoplasms.

Mucoepidermoid Tumour

This tumour is characterized by the presence of squamous cells, mucus-secreting cells, and cells of an intermediate type. The relative proportions of these cells vary. When squamous cells predominate the tumour tends to be solid: when mucous cells predominate soft tumours which have cystic spaces occur. Although the proportions of these cell types may vary from tumour to tumour, both mucus secretion and the presence of squamous cells should be demonstrable before a tumour is accorded to this category. Stromal variation is not a feature of muco-epidermoid tumours. The degree of cellular differentiation together with the behavioural pattern varies, and although the less well-differentiated tumours tend to be more aggressive and may metastasize, this is not always the case. Although these tumours should always be considered as potentially malignant, the majority pursue a benign course and with adequate surgical excision can be considered as curable lesions.

Acinic Cell Tumour

The neoplasm comprises cells similar to the serous acinar cells of salivary glands. The tumour has a predilection for the parotid gland. The tumour consists of round or polygonal cells, the cystoplasm of which displays a varying degree of basophilia and granularity. Acinar-like formations are characteristic, although solid sheets of tumour cells may be present. On rare occasions, despite a benign histological appearance, the acinic-cell tumour may infiltrate locally or metastasize.

Carcinomas

Malignant disease of the salivary glands is fortunately relatively rare. Histologically, five types are recognized, as follows:

Adenoid cystic carcinoma. This infiltrative malignant neoplasm comprises tumour cells which are polygonal in shape, display basophilia and aggregate together to form a characteristic cribriform or cylindromatous appearance. The tumour cells form duct-like structures enclosing alcian blue positive material which is in continuity with the supporting connective tissue. In some regions, myoepithelial cells may proliferate, giving a lace-like pattern to that region of the tumour. A more solid variant may recur. The tumour is not encapsulated and grows slowly, having a proclivity to invade neuro-vascular sheaths and metastasize late.

Adenocarcinoma. The adenocarcinoma is a malignant epithelial tumour which histo-pathologically exhibits some tubule or papillary glandular formation. Those features which characterize the pleomorphic adenoma are absent. As in other salivary neoplasms, variation in histological appearance is common. Cystic or papillary formations, oxyphilic change and tubule formation may be observed.

Epidermoid carcinoma. This tumour is characterized by malignant epithelial cells of salivary origin which form keratin or exhibit intercellular bridges. Mucus secretion is absent.

Undifferentiated carcinoma. These tumours, although recognizable as malignant lesions of epithelial origin, are too poorly differentiated to be placed in any other category. In some of the tumours admitted to this group, spindle- or spheroidal-shaped cells may predominate.

Carcinoma in pleomorphic adenoma. In some areas this tumour shows histopathological features which are characteristic of pleomorphic adenoma, whilst in other areas definite evidence of malignancy is present. Thus, cytological changes appropriate to carcinoma, together with evidence of invasive growth, will be present in such lesions.

Aetiology

No substantial evidence has been produced to implicate a virus, a carcinogen or preceding disease of the glands as a causal agent for the development of salivary neoplasia in man. The exact cell of origin of the individual salivary-gland-tumour types remains unknown at the present time. It seems reasonable to conclude that a duct cell is the principal cell type in the majority of tumours. The role of the myoepithelial cell in salivary neoplasms, especially with regard to its inductive effect upon supporting tissues, is receiving attention at the present time. The changes occurring in connective tissue in the pleomorphic adenoma, for example, are judged to represent metaplasia rather than neoplasia.

Diagnosis

The diagnosis of salivary gland neoplasia depends largely upon clinical appearances and behaviour, together with histological examination of a biopsy specimen. Biopsy techniques and other tests of gland function which may aid the diagnosis and allow differentiation from other salivary lesions are described elsewhere in this text.

Treatment

The treatment of the vast majority of salivary gland neoplasms is effected best by surgical excision. The pleomorphic adenoma is relatively radio-resistant. Where there is evidence of metastasis, however, a broad oncological approach must be taken. Thus, excision of regional lymph nodes, chemotherapy and/or irradiation may be indicated. Possible complications of surgery to the salivary glands include facial nerve damage, gustatory sweating and fistula formation. Such complications, fortunately, are rare.

SJÖGREN'S SYNDROME

Introduction

Sjögren's syndrome consists of the triad of xerostomia, keratoconjunctivitis sicca and a connective tissue disorder, usually rheumatoid arthritis but occasionally systemic lupus erythematosus, progressive systemic sclerosis, polyarteritis nodosa or polymyositis. The presence of two of the three main components is generally sufficient for the diagnosis of the syndrome. The term 'sicca syndrome' is used when only xerostomia and keratoconjunctivitis are present. In Sjögren's syndrome, a preponderance of female patients, especially in the post-menopausal age group, is consistently noted, though the presence of this disorder in adolescents has been reported. The frequency with which Sjögren's syndrome is recognized depends upon the awareness of the examiner who first sees the patient. Several studies, indeed, suggest that the syndrome may be a relatively common disorder. These factors, together with the presence of regional rheumatology centres, may account for the apparently high frequency of the disease in areas such as Bethesda, Maryland, some Scandinavian countries and in Glasgow. With regard to the incidence of the disease, it is to be noted that, among the connective tissue diseases, Sjögren's syndrome takes second place only to rheumatoid arthritis.

The suggested 'autoimmune' association and the spectrum of benign-to-malignant lymphoproliferation in the syndrome are well documented. Although the cause of the disease remains unknown, it seems likely that a combination of genetic, immunological, viral and/or environmental factors may play a role in the pathogenesis. It is clear that if we could understand the basic mechanisms concerned in Sjögren's syndrome, aetiological factors in rheumatoid arthritis and lymphoid neoplasia might be revealed, and this accounts for the considerable interest in Sjögren's syndrome during recent years.

Keratoconjunctivitis sicca and rheumatoid arthritis are readily diagnosed by well-defined criteria. Xerostomia is a common clinical complaint with a multiplicity of causes and predisposing factors.

Although much attention has been directed towards the salivary glands and their secretions in Sjögren's syndrome, the salivary gland dysfunction is less well defined than the other components of the disorder. In addition to clinical studies, investigative procedures include salivary flow-rate estimation, sialography and labial salivary gland biopsy. Furthermore, the salivary glands and their secretions have been studied in the laboratory using the techniques of serology, immunopathology, biochemistry, microbiology and electron microscopy.

Clinical Features

Xerostomia

Patients should be carefully questioned regarding the history and duration of xerostomia and of associated oral and pharyngeal symptoms. Decreased salivation, difficulty in swallowing and mastication, increased fluid intake, abnormalities of taste and smell, oral mucosal soreness, ulceration and fissuring are common symptoms. The oral mucous membranes are described as being dry, smooth and shiny (Figure 14.3). Lingual changes (Figure 14.4), varying from slight reddening with mild fissuring to severe lobulation, have been reported. In patients with natural teeth, a rapidly progressive caries is noted, whilst those with dentures often have difficulty with retention. It is important, of course, to exclude other causes of xerostomia, such as drugs, irradiation and anaemia.

Salivary Gland Enlargement

Salivary gland enlargement was present in 30 per cent of the cases reported by Rauch (1959). Our experience over a 10-year period has been that, although a history of gland enlargement is elicited from approximately 30 per cent of patients, its presence is clinically apparent in only 15 per cent of cases (Figure 14.5). Most studies agree that the swelling is bilateral and that the parotid glands are more commonly affected. The differential diagnosis of salivary gland enlargement must include infections, neoplasia, drugs and other systemic disease such as diabetes mellitus.

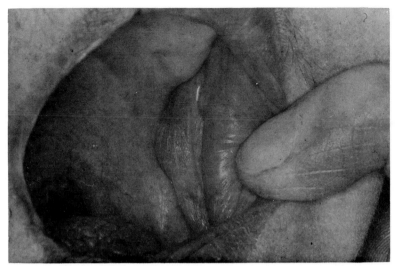

Figure 14.3. Extreme oral dryness, atrophic mucosae and lobulated tongue in patient with longstanding Sjögren's syndrome.

Relative Value of Salivary Gland Function Tests in Clinical Diagnosis

There is, as yet, no entirely satisfactory test of gland dysfunction in Sjögren's syndrome. Parotid salivary flow-rate measurement has the disadvantage of examining the secretion from only one gland and no statement can be made concerning total or whole salivary volume. However, measurement of total mixed saliva is less accurate and requires collection by drainage or spitting, which can be unpleasant for the patient. The parotid glands make the main contribution to whole saliva on stimulation. For these reasons and also because, as mentioned above, the parotid glands are the most

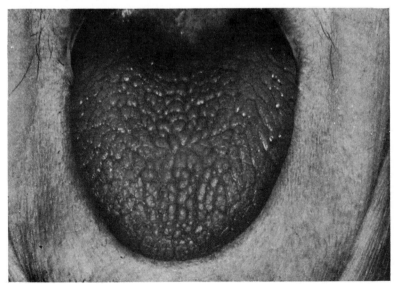

Figure 14.4. Severe lobulation and fissuring of tongue in patient with Sjögren's syndrome and xerostomia of 22 years' duration.

commonly involved in Sjögren's syndrome, we have favoured measurement of parotid flow rates to that of mixed saliva.

The demonstration of subnormal stimulated parotid salivary flow rates is the most sensitive index of salivary dysfunction in Sjögren's syndrome, followed in order of sensitivity by labial salivary gland biopsy, which reveals focal lymphocytic adenitis, and sialography.

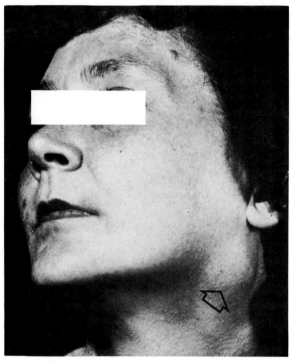

Figure 14.5. Firm, painless swelling of left parotid salivary gland in a patient with sicca syndrome.

In our clinics, in order to diagnose Sjögren's syndrome with salivary gland involvement, the following steps are undertaken when a patient presents with xerostomia and possible Sjögren's syndrome:

1. A careful clinical examination and history is taken to exclude all other causes of xerostomia or salivary gland enlargement.
2. Swabs and smears are taken from tongue, palate, buccal mucosa and fitting surface of dentures.
3. Maximum stimulated (10 per cent citric acid) parotid salivary flow rates are measured.
4. A labial salivary gland biopsy is performed to confirm the nature of the disease process.
5. Sialography and/or scintiscanning (Tc^{99m} pertechnetate) are undertaken if the flow-rate values are equivocal.
6. The ophthalmological and general medical examinations including haematological and serological work-up, are best undertaken by ophthalmologists and rheumatologists. Serological studies should include salivary duct antibody, anti-nuclear factor, rheumatoid factor, anti-thyroid, DNA antibody titres and mitochondrial antibody estimations.

Treatment

The treatment, both local and general, of the distressing oral symptoms of Sjögren's syndrome, requires a broad approach. It is important that the oral mucous membranes be kept as moist as possible. Glycerine lozenges, methylcellulose (2 per cent solution) as a lubricant may be of benefit to some patients. A mouthwash containing citric acid (25 g), essence of lemon (40 ml) and glycerine (made up to 2 litres) has been used with some success in our clinics. Patients should be encouraged to increase their fluid intake and to take sips of water throughout the day, especially during meals, whilst oral hygiene should be scrupulous. Local infections such as candidosis should be detected and treated with appropriate drug therapy. Salivary gland enlargement usually subsides but painful recalcitrant swellings may be treated with analgesics and anti-biotics. Irradiation is contra-indicated in view of the known association of Sjögren's syndrome and lymphoid neoplasia.

Systemic therapy, such as corticosteroids, do not improve the oral symptoms. The management of keratoconjunctivitis sicca with lubricating agents such as 1 per cent methylcellulose is essential if long-term complications, such as corneal ulceration, are to be avoided.

LYMPHOEPITHELIAL LESION

Lymphoepithelial lesion, or Mikulicz's disease, has many similarities to Sjögren's syndrome, not least of which is an identical histopathology. However, the condition lacks the systemic involvement of Sjögren's syndrome and there is value in considering the diseases as separate entities at the present time. Lymphoepithelial lesion should be distinguished from Mikulicz's syndrome, which is salivary enlargement of known cause, such as sarcoidosis.

SIALOSIS

Sialosis is the term which is used to describe a non-inflammatory, non-neoplastic recurrent bilateral swelling of the salivary glands. The parotid glands are much more commonly affected than the submandibular, sublingual or minor salivary glands. Although the cause is not known, the condition is associated with numerous other diseases, such as endocrine abnormalities and nutritional deficiencies, and may follow the ingestion of various drugs. Regardless of the numerous associated conditions in sialosis there is a striking uniformity in the clinical appearances, histopathological changes and salivary enzyme constituents in affected individuals.

Clinical Features

The onset of salivary gland enlargement is slow, generally painless and unaccompanied by the signs or symptoms of inflammation. Multiglandular involvement, usually sym-metrical, is a characteristic feature. Women are more commonly affected. It is of interest that in the majority of cases the enlargement involves principally the pre-auricular portion of the parotid gland.

Diagnosis

The elevation of potassium in saliva of affected individuals from 25 mmol/l to 35—50 mmol/l may be an important diagnostic aid. Sialography reveals a duct structure of normal architecture and there appears to be little alteration in stimulated salivary flow-rate values. The histology of sialosis is characterized by serous acinar-cell hypertrophy, oedema of the interstitial supporting tissue and atrophy of the striated ducts. The cytoplasm of the hypertrophic serous cells is more mucoid and less granular than normal. The lesion may progress to a lipomatosis of the affected glands.

These general features, then, characterize sialosis. The majority of cases reported have been related to hormonal disturbances, chiefly ovarian, thyroid and pancreatic dysfunction, and to malnutrition, liver cirrhosis and chronic alcoholism. Drug-induced sialosis in experimental animals following the administration of various adrenergic and cholinergic drugs is well known whilst, in human beings, parotid enlargement has been noted in patients taking various medications such as phenylbutazone.

Classification

The various sialoses may be classified according to their clinical association as hormonal, neurohumoral, dysenzymatic, malnutritional and drug induced.

Hormonal Sialosis

Sialosis may occur as a result of dysfunction of the sex hormones and has been described following ovariectomy, in gynaecomastia, during pregnancy and at the time of menopause. Raised potassium levels in resting saliva appear to be a constant feature in these conditions.

Bilateral parotid enlargement has been described in diabetes mellitus (Figure 14.6). The reduced flow-rate values which have been reported in diabetes, together with the increased susceptibility to infection, make sialadenitis a common complication.

In man, iodide is concentrated in saliva to many times the plasma level and there is evidence to suggest that the site of concentration is the salivary ducts. Iodide is extensively used in expectorants and asthma preparations, in the preoperative treatment of hyperthyroidism and as a radio-opaque substance for diagnostic radiography. Toxic reactions including enlargement of the salivary glands may be a complication of iodide administration. Salivary enlargement is usually associated with long-term administration of iodide although the condition may develop suddenly.

Neurohumoral Sialosis

Sialosis may follow disease or irritation of the autonomic nervous system either peripherally or centrally. Bilateral parotid enlargement in patients suffering from gastric spasm or bronchial asthma has been described. A small group of patients with severe psychic disturbances who displayed adiposity, oligomenorrhoea and parotid enlargement has also been described.

Dysenzymatic Sialosis

Hepatogenic sialosis affecting the parotid glands is commonly observed in patients with alcoholic cirrhosis. Sialosis, however, may occur in alcoholics in the absence of cirrhosis or in cirrhosis due to other causes. Biopsy of affected glands has shown marked acinar oedema to be a notable feature. Chronic secondary infection is present in nearly one half of patients. Nephrogenic sialosis appears to be exceedingly rare. Parotid enlargement and increased parotid flow rates in patients with chronic relapsing pancreatitis have been reported. Biopsies from these patients revealed hypertrophy of the acinar cells and no apparent change in the duct elements. An association between recurrent parotid swelling, arterial hypertension and pancreatitis has also been reported. Salivary gland enlargement, together with stomatitis, may be present in cases of uraemia, though resolution follows renal dialysis.

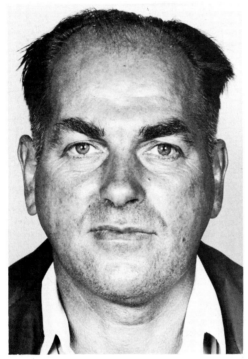

Figure 14.6. Bilateral parotid enlargement in a patient with diabetes mellitus.

Malnutritional Sialosis

Soft painless enlargement of the salivary glands may occur in nutritional deficiency states, especially where there is a qualitative and quantitative lack of protein in the diet. Children appear to be more commonly affected in those regions where malnutrition is a problem.

Bilateral, asymptomatic parotid gland enlargement may be associated with prolonged starch ingestion.

Drug-induced Sialosis

Parotid enlargement has been noted in patients taking medications such as phenylbutazone. The anti-inflammatory effect of phenylbutazone drugs had led to their use in rheumatoid arthritis and allied conditions. The pharmacology is poorly understood although the drug probably acts by decreasing capillary permeability. Adverse reactions and allergic responses to phenylbutazone drugs may occur and it is possible that salivary gland enlargement may reflect this phenomenon. Xerostomia and signs and symptoms of acute sialadenitis may be accompanying features. These reactions respond to the cessation of drug administration. Antibiotics and/or corticosteroid therapy may be of value in the treatment. Iodide-containing compounds, thiouracil, catecholamines and sulphonamides have also been reported as inducing sialosis.

Drug-induced sialosis in experimental animals may follow the administration of various adrenergic and cholinergic drugs. Administration of isoprenaline (isoproterenol), a β-adrenergic drug, produces a marked enlargement of the salivary glands of the rat and mouse.

In summary, sialosis appears to be a well defined clinical entity. Although predisposing factors may vary, a final common pathway may operate in each case.

FURTHER READING

Chisholm, D. M. & Mason, D. K. (1973) Salivary gland function in Sjögren's syndrome: a review. *British Dental Journal,* **135,** 393.

Evans, R. W. & Cruickshank, A. H. (1970) *Epithelial Tumours of the Salivary Glands.* Philadelphia, London, Toronto: W. B. Saunders.

Rauch, S. (1959) *Die Speicheldrüsen des Munschen.* Stuttgart: Georg Thieme Verlag.

Shearn, M. A. (1971) *Sjögren's Syndrome.* Philadelphia, London, Toronto: W. B. Saunders.

Thackray, A. C. (1972) *International Histological Classification of Tumours. Histological Typing of Salivary Gland Tumours.* Geneva: World Health Organization.

Thackray, A. C. & Lucas, R. B. (1974) *Tumors of the Major Salivary Glands,* Atlas of Tumor Pathology, 2nd series, fascicle 10. Washington, D.C.: Armed Forces Institute of Pathology.

DISEASE OF BONE, CONNECTIVE TISSUE AND JOINT

chapter 15

Development, Structure and Function

The Connective Tissues
Bone
The Temporomandibular Joint

THE CONNECTIVE TISSUES

The connective tissues are the most widely distributed and most abundant of all the body's tissue elements and are involved in most of its functional activities. They are continuous throughout, and include tendons, fascia, ligaments, joint capsules, septa and organ capsules, interstitial tissue, cartilage and bone, and adipose and mucous tissues. All these are derived from the primitive mesodermal tissue, which in the adult persists to some extent in the loose connective tissues and newly-formed granulation tissue which follows injury to a part.

Despite the fact that the connective tissue forms such a large proportion of the body tissues, surprisingly little is known about its functions. Mechanical support and protection are among the most important functions and have been long recognized. The smooth interaction of the parts of the body is facilitated by lubrication of ground substance components. Energy stores of fat and protein are released from the connective tissues for use in response to hormonal stimulus. Since connective tissue is interposed between blood vessels and epithelially derived structures, it necessarily has an important function as an organ of transport of both essential nutrients and metabolic waste products. Antibody production, together with the inflammatory process and reparative potential, establish the connective tissues as the seat of the most important defence systems in the body.

BONE

Structure

Bone is a mineralized or calcified connective tissue by virtue of the deposition of inorganic mineral rich in calcium within the intercellular collagen mucopolysaccharide matrix.

171

Adult bone is readily divided into compact bone, composed of solid mineralized matrix and coarse cancellous bone which is spongy in character, the matrix framework being obvious to the naked eye. During bone development, the initial fine cancellous structure is gradually remodelled into either compact or coarse cancellous bone or removed altogether in the formation of a marrow space (Figure 15.1).

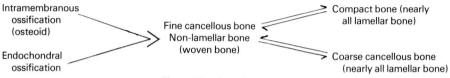

Figure 15.1. Bone formation.

Bone matrix has an organic component consisting of collagen fibres aggregated into fibres and fibre bundles within a ground substance containing mucopolysaccharide. This organic component comprises one-third of the dry weight of bone matrix, whilst an inorganic component consisting mainly of calcium phosphate in microcrystalline form makes up the remaining two-thirds. Bone matrix is lamellar or non-lamellar, depending on whether or not it exhibits a laminated appearance when viewed in sections with polarized light. Non-lamellar bone is often called 'woven bone'. In adult bone, whether it is of the compact or coarse cancellous type, the matrix is mostly of the lamellar variety.

The bone cells are a closely related group which includes osteocytes, osteoblasts, osteoclasts and osteoprogenitor cells. The osteoprogenitor cell is the fundamental cell, and may be in a dormant state, or undergoing mitotic division or transforming into an osteoblast or osteoclast. These cells are normally confined to the vicinity of bone but under abnormal conditions may appear in almost any connective tissue and initiate heterotopic bone formation. Osteoblasts produce bone matrix and do not divide. Many become trapped in matrix, becoming osteocytes, whilst others may revert to the osteoprogenitor type. Osteoclasts are actively involved in bone matrix resorption and are considered to arise from fusion of osteoprogenitor cells. Osteocytes are thought to regulate the flow of minerals and nutrients between bone and blood, and thus maintain the bone matrix around them.

Bone is a richly vascular tissue, with the direction of flow, especially of smaller vessels, being towards the periosteum. The periosteum is a fibrous membrane which ensheaths bone, except at cartilage-covered surfaces and where tendons and ligaments are attached. The periosteum functions as a muscle attachment, a vascular supporting tissue and also as an agent in bone growth and repair. Adult periosteum presumably contains dormant osteoprogenitor cells which respond to a variety of stimuli by enlargement, multiplication and conversion into osteoblasts or osteoclasts. Bone marrow is the soft red or yellow tissue occupying the macroscopically visible cavities in a fresh bone. It comprises a meshwork of reticular tissue, blood vessels (especially venous sinusoids) and either colonies of developing blood cells or large fat cells. Reticulum cells readily transform into osteoprogenitor cells.

Ossification (Bone Formation, Osteogenesis)

The production of fine cancellous bone from precursor fibrous and cartilaginous tissues is achieved by either primary intramembranous ossification or primary endochondral ossification.

Primary intramembranous ossification characterizes the early ossification in the face and skull as well as general periosteal, tendinous and ligamentous ossification. A fibrous framework with vascular interstices is first formed. Through the action of osteoblasts evolved from the local connective tissue cell population, this framework is converted into bone matrix. This involves, in addition, the formation of more collagenous fibres and cement and the deposition of hydroxyapatite. The matrix is called osteoid before it is calcified. The primary membrane bone which results has the form of a fine cancellous framework of non-lamellar bone matrix whose interstices are occupied by osteoblasts, osteoprogenitor cells and wide capillaries. Osteocytes are buried within the matrix whilst fibre bundles are incorporated in the osteoid and matrix. Primary endochondral ossification takes place at centres of ossification in the cartilage and at the cartilaginous ends of growing bones. Cartilage matrix formation is followed by calcification. Cell death occurs, leaving a honeycomb of calcified cartilage matrix. Invasion by osteoprogenitor cells and blood vessels results in resorption of portions of the calcified cartilage network, allowing the deposition of bone matrix by osteoblasts. The first matrix contains fine uniform bundles of fibres. The fine cancellous cartilage bone differs from fine cancellous membrane bone in that it has calcified cartilage remnants in its matrix and by the regular arrangement of its fibre bundles. In both forms of fine cancellous bone, osteoclastic resorption and osteoblastic deposition together alter the texture and structure of the matrix, such that compact or coarse cancellous forms result with an increasing content of lamellar bone.

Bone Matrix Formation

It is considered that osteoblasts secrete collagen molecules (tropocollagen), mucopolysaccharides and glycoproteins. Outside the cells, the collagen molecules aggregate into fibrils and these in turn form into fibres and fibre bundles. Fibre orientation appears to be influenced by osteoblastic activity.

Development and Growth of Bones

In essence, the development and growth of a bone begins with the formation and growth of a fibrous, or a cartilaginous and fibrous model. This is followed by the formation and growth of a primary bony model within and at the expense of the original model. The emergence of the definitive adult bone through remodelling of the primary bone model is followed by further remodelling which is concerned with the maintenance, adaptation and repair of the adult bone. In most bones in fetal life, ossification begins at points called primary centres of ossification, and most of the bony tissue of the adult skeleton is formed as a result of growth at these centres. Outside the skull, secondary centres of ossification appear and grow into bony epiphyses. Bone laid down at centres of ossification is of the fine cancellous variety. Remodelling of the developing bony mass results in either a more compact or a more coarsely cancellous type of bone.

THE TEMPOROMANDIBULAR JOINT

Development

The mandibular joint develops in the condensation of mesenchyme cells, separating the developing squamous portion of the temporal bone from the condylar cartilage which forms on the dorsal surface of the developing mandibular ramus. The mandibular condensation maps out the shape of the condyle. Intramembranous ossification commences in the 30-mm CR (crown—rump) embryo in temporal bone which, at this stage, is widely separated from the mandibular portion of the joint. Differentiation of the cartilage of the mandibular condyle at the 50-mm CR stage serves to bring the temporal and mandibular elements closer together. Growth is rapid and at the 65-mm CR stage the interarticular space is narrow and contains a thin strip of tissue destined to become the articular disc. This tissue is connected to the lateral pterygoid muscle from its first appearance. The condylar cartilage forms a cone-shaped mass and growth advances by apposition. The communication between the growing joint and middle ear persists until the 270—300-mm CR stage. The joint capsule is usually well formed by a condensation of surrounding mesenchyme by the 180-mm CR stage. The articular eminence is not well formed at birth and begins to assume its characteristic form only with the establishment of the primary dentition. In the temporal region, small areas of secondary cartilage contribute to growth but are not present by the time of birth.

Structure

The temporomandibular joint is a condylar joint between the articular tubercle and the anterior portion of the mandibular fossa of the temporal bone above and the head of the mandible below. Both articular surfaces are covered by a layer of dense white fibrocartilage. An articular disc divides the joint into an upper and lower cavity. The joint capsule is attached above to the margins of the glenoid fossa and articular eminence and below to the articular margin of the head of the condyle. Collateral ligaments, the temporomandibular and sphenomandibular, strengthen the capsule and limit condylar movement. The capsule is more fully developed posteriorly where it comes into contact with the articular disc. The articular disc is an oval plate of fibrous tissue, the upper surface of which is concavoconvex from the front backwards. In front, the disc is attached to the tendon of the lateral pterygoid muscle whilst its circumference is attached to the capsule.

Blood is supplied from the deep auricular branch of the internal maxillary artery. The pterygoid plexus of veins drains the joint. The nerve supply to the joint is provided by the mandibular division of the trigeminal nerve through its auriculotemporal branch.

Function

The movements of the mandible comprise depression and elevation, lateral, protrusive and retrusive movements. Contraction of the lateral pterygoid muscles initiates jaw opening from the position of centric occlusion. Co-ordinated relaxation of the masseter, temporalis and medial pterygoid and contraction of the anterior belly of the digastric and suprahyoid muscles effects this movement. Jaw closure is achieved by contraction of masseter, temporalis and medial pterygoid with relaxation of the lateral pterygoid. Rotational movement is achieved when the condyle on one side is held in the articular fossa by muscle contraction on that side. Protrusion and retrusion are achieved by contraction or relaxation of the medial and lateral pterygoid whilst tonic contraction of the masseter is maintained.

FURTHER READING

Bloom, W. & Fawcett, D. W. (1964) *A Textbook of Histology,* 8th ed. Philadelphia, London, Toronto: W. B. Saunders.
Scott, J. H. & Symons, N. B. B. (1961) *Introduction to Dental Anatomy,* 3rd ed. Edinburgh, London: E. & S. Livingstone.

chapter 16

Bone Disease

Introduction
Diagnosis
Developmental Lesions of the Jaws
Inflammatory Disease of Bone
Metabolic Diseases of the Jaws
Fibro-osseous Lesions
Tumours and Tumour-like Swellings of Bone

INTRODUCTION

The bones of the face are subject to disease which may be generalized or local in nature. In generalized disease of the skeleton, the maxilla and/or the mandible may be the first bones to show clinical or radiographic evidence of disease; for example Paget's disease of bone, or osteitis fibrosa. The recognition of these early changes is a fundamental aspect of the practice of oral medicine. The changes which take place in the jaw bones in these systemic diseases may lead to symptoms suggesting a localized condition, such as difficulty with dentures, looseness of teeth, localized swelling and facial pain. In some instances, the condition may be confined to one bone of the face; for example, fibrous dysplasia of the monostotic type.

The fact that the jaw bones support teeth and may contain epithelial remnants of tooth development accounts for the high incidence of localized infection in the jaws, such as dento-alveolar abscess and inflammatory cyst formation. In addition, tumours of odontogenic origin almost always involve bone and present as bony swellings accompanied by radiographic change.

Metabolic disease of bone may lead to profound biochemical changes in serum, many of which are characteristic or pathognomonic for the condition.

DIAGNOSIS

The diagnosis of bone diseases of the jaws is established by a combination of clinical, radiological and histopathological investigation, supplemented when necessary by biochemical and haematological studies. These are now considered.

175

Radiology

This has a role of the utmost importance. The relevant radiological information should always be available to the clinician and to the histopathologist, and group discussion by those concerned in diagnosis and treatment is to be encouraged. Radiographs permit assessment of the form and structure of the normal elements; of bone destruction as indicated by abnormal radiolucency and the margin of this radiolucency, whether rounded or irregular and indistinct; of abnormal ossification and calcification causing opacity; and of abnormality in the structure of bone.

Histopathology

The histopathology of diseased bone is often, though not always, essential for precise diagnosis. Bone biopsies may be taken using a variety of chisels and drills. The bone is usually fixed in formalin and decalcified before paraffin-embedding and section-cutting. Microscopic examination is usually made by transmitted illumination and by polarizing techniques.

Biochemical and Haematological Studies

The estimation of calcium, phosphorus, alkaline phosphatase and acid phosphatase in serum is important in the diagnosis of diseases such as Paget's disease of bone and osteitis fibrosa.

Plasma and urinary proteins, urinary catecholamines and bone-marrow cytology, together with haematological investigation, may be of value in individual cases.

DEVELOPMENTAL LESIONS OF THE JAWS

Facial Clefts

Facial clefts occur as a failure of fusion in embryonic processes. Cleft lips may be complete or incomplete and approximately 80 per cent are unilaterally affected. Males are affected in 55 to 60 per cent of cases. The association of cleft lips and cleft alveolus occurs in 70 per cent of cases. Cleft palate may be total or the cleft may affect only the uvula — bifid uvula.

Facial clefts are sometimes accompanied by other defects such as congenital heart disease and polydactylia. The tendency to such defects may be inherited, but diet, trauma and infections have been implicated in some cases.

Surgical treatment is employed, with early soft-tissue closure followed by hard-tissue closure at a later date, supported by dental therapy involving specialist orthodontic and restorative services.

Fissural Non-odontogenic Cysts

Developmental cysts arise from inclusion of epithelial remnants within bone at the time of fusion of embryonic processes. They include median mandibular, medial palatal, nasopalatine and globulomaxillary cysts and all usually require surgical removal.

Median mandibular and median palatal cysts arise from epithelium entrapped between the processes which meet to form the mandible and palate during development. They may be so large as to produce a visible swelling but are often discovered by chance on radiology in connection with some other complaint. These cysts have a fibrous tissue wall and are lined by stratified squamous epithelium. Treatment is by surgical removal.

Nasopalatine cysts are found in the incisive canal and arise from remnants of the nasopalatine duct which joins the mouth and nose during development. These cysts are not uncommon and present as rounded swellings or are found incidentally on radiographic examination of the anterior part of the hard palate. Occasionally, the cysts are secondarily infected with all the signs and symptoms of an acute infection. The cysts have a thick fibrous wall in which large blood vessels and nerves, present because of the site of the cyst, are usually identified. The cyst lining is of stratified squamous, ciliated columnar or cuboidal epithelium. Surgical removal is the treatment of choice.

Globulomaxillary cysts are found between the upper lateral incisor and canine teeth where the globular part of the median nasal process and the maxillary process meet during development of the face. The cyst is usually discovered as an incidental finding on dental radiography, where it shows as a pear-shaped radiolucency between and separating the roots of the teeth. The wall is composed of fibrous tissue and the cyst is lined by stratified squamous or by columnar ciliated epithelium. Treatment is by surgical excision.

Developmental Odontogenic Cysts

(a) Primordial cyst (keratocyst)
(b) Dentigerous cyst

The primordial cyst (keratocyst) is a developmental odontogenic cyst arising in the tooth-bearing areas of the jaws. The most common site is the mandibular molar region and, again, the lesion extends into the ramus. In some instances, the cyst may form in an area where a tooth has failed to develop.

Radiographically, the primordial cyst may show a unilocular or multilocular pattern. The lining epithelium is thin, rarely exceeding five cells in thickness and having no rete pegs. The keratinization of the epithelium is usually of the parakeratotic type, although orthokeratosis may be noted. Separate small cysts may develop in the connective tissue capsule. Primordial cysts have a marked tendency to recur following excision, excision being the treatment of choice.

Multiple primordial cysts may be associated with other abnormalities such as multiple naevoid basal cell carcinoma and bifid rib, and the condition is known as the Gorlin and Goltz syndrome.

The dentigerous cyst is one which grows in the enamel organ of an unerupted tooth. This developmental cyst is most commonly found in relation to the mandibular third molar, the maxillary canine and third molar, and the mandibular second premolar. Radiographically, a well-defined radiolucency is noted in relation to the crown of the tooth. A thin stratified squamous epithelial lining is present.

Osteogenesis Imperfecta

This disorder, inherited through an autosomal dominant gene of variable penetrance, is an abnormality in the formation of collagen which results in an inadequate bone matrix. Osteogenesis imperfecta constitutes a spectrum of disease, ranging from a lethal form to a condition of mild thinning and fragility of bones. Blue sclera and otosclerosis may accompany the disease, but are not an invariable accompaniment.

Clinically, a history of multiple fractures is usually elicited. The oral manifestations include thinning of the cortical bone of the jaws and defective formation of enamel and dentine (Figure 16.1). In affected teeth, the coronal portion is small, the roots are reduced in length and breadth and the pulp cavities are frequently obliterated. Currently, no effective treatment exists.

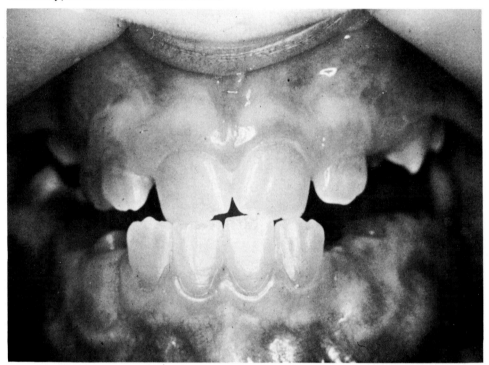

Figure 16.1. Dentogenesis imperfecta occurring in a case of osteogenesis imperfecta.

Osteopetrosis (Marble Bone Disease)

The aetiology of this condition is unknown. The clinical features are those of generalized bone density. Thus, fractures, infections and cranial nerve compression may complicate the picture. The disease may affect patients early in life and, in these circumstances, is highly progressive. Onset later in life is less dramatic. Radiographically, the extreme density of bone is reflected in increased radiopacity. An increased dental caries rate may be noted. Serum calcium and phosphorus levels are within the normal ranges. Obliteration of marrow space may induce anaemia. Care should be taken during extraction of the teeth since there are risks of jaw fracture, post-extraction infection and delay in healing.

Cleidocranial Dysostosis

The aetiology of this unusual, rare condition is unknown, although a hereditary factor may be present.

Clinically, a variety of skeletal abnormalities is observed, including absence or poor development of the clavicle, frontal and nasal bones and abnormality and delayed eruption of the permanent dentition. Thus, the patient may present with nasal bridge depression, and median frontal bone furrowing and lateral frontal bulging are evident. Intra-orally, the primary dentition is often retained. Supernumerary teeth are commonly seen and dentigerous cysts may occur. In dentistry, such cases present problems of management from both conservative and surgical points of view (Figure 16.2).

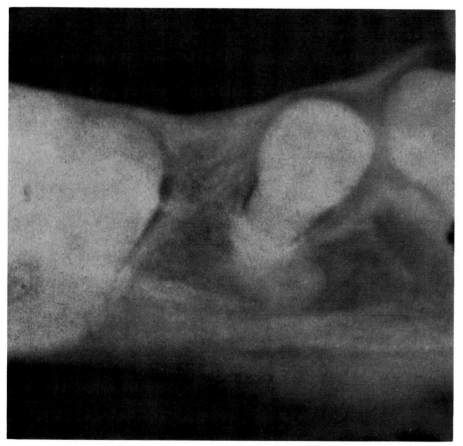

Figure 16.2. Gross dental abnormalities in a case of cleidocranial dysostosis.

INFLAMMATORY DISEASE OF BONE

Osteomyelitis of the Jaws

This is an inflammation of the soft tissues within bone. In the majority of cases *Staphylococcus aureus* is the causative organism although, rarely, *Actinomyces israelii* may be implicated. The infection reaches the bone from nearby infection; for example, in association with the teeth or with the maxillary antrum, by direct implantation following trauma or by the blood stream from a distant site. In infancy, the maxilla is more commonly involved than the mandible, while in children and in adults the reverse is the case. It is important to stress that osteomyelitis is relatively rare nowadays due to effective chemotherapy of infections in the jaws.

The following types of osteomyelitis will be described: acute and chronic suppurative osteomyelitis; chronic focal, and chronic diffuse, sclerosing osteomyelitis; and chronic osteomyelitis with proliferating periostitis.

Acute Suppurative Osteomyelitis

This is usually painful and accompanied by an elevation of temperature. There may be numbness of the lip if the inferior dental nerve is involved. Radiographically, no change is observed in the early lesion whilst later stages are characterized by patchy radiolucencies. The formation of pus, necrotic bone and sequestrae are features of both. Surgical drainage and curettage are complemented by antibiotic therapy.

Chronic Suppurative Osteomyelitis

This results from a longstanding infection. Radiographically, radiolucent areas are present. Sequestrae are formulated: these are portions of non-vital bone which are supported by vital bone at their periphery. Treatment is similar to that for acute infection.

Chronic Focal Sclerosing Osteomyelitis

This form is usually noted in patients under 20 years of age and the third molar region is a common site. The condition is generally symptomless although, radiographically, an area of radiopacity is noted near the root apices of a tooth which shows pulpal inflammation or necrosis.

Chronic Diffuse Sclerosing Osteomyelitis

This variant is usually observed in older people, commonly those between 40 and 50 years of age. The lesion represents a proliferative response to periapical infection. The condition is usually symptomless and, radiographically, diffuse sclerotic areas are noted, often in an edentulous mandible.

Chronic Osteomyelitis with Proliferative Periostitis

Usually, this type is seen in the mandible, associated with dental caries with pulpal and periapical sequelae. Proliferation of periosteal tissues is accompanied by irregular bone deposition on the superficial surface of bone, producing a visible swelling. Offending teeth should be extracted. The disease tends to resolve with bone remodelling taking place. It should be noted that any infection of the jaws in children may involve tooth germs and/or bone growth centres, leading to dental or bone malformation and deformity.

Treatment of osteomyelitis. The combination of chemotherapeutic agents and surgical curettage is usually effective. Clindamycin and lincomycin are effective antibiotics in recalcitrant cases.

Necrosis of the Jaws

Chemical Necrosis

This is rarely seen now although, in the past, arsenic used as an endodontic agent and yellow phosphorus used in industry gave rise, on occasion, to necrosis of bone in exposed individuals.

Irradiation Necrosis

This may follow radiotherapy for orofacial neoplasia. Severe pain is a feature. Histologically, the changes are those of degeneration, ranging from oedema to necrosis with thickening of the walls of blood vessels as a characteristic feature. Surgical treatment is indicated in most cases.

Dento-alveolar Abscess

This is an acute suppurative process, associated with teeth, in which a periapical or periodontal abscess develops. The cause is generally necrosis and infection of the pulp, resulting from dental caries or trauma. A variety of organisms may be recovered, including *Streptococcus viridans*, *Streptococcus haemolyticus* and *Staphylococcus aureus*.

The onset of abscess formation is heralded by severe, throbbing pain, often easily localized by the patient. The pus in the abscess drains through the root canal or tracks along the line of least resistance into the mouth, the maxillary antrum, posteriorly to the tissue spaces of the neck, or to the skin. A marked swelling of soft tissue usually occurs, associated with a reduction in pain intensity. There may be regional lymph node enlargement, pyrexia and malaise.

Radiographically, the primary acute lesion does not show a radiolucent area. Radiolucency, together with sclerosing osteitis, characterize longstanding lesions.

Treatment is a surgical matter, usually requiring extraction of the offending tooth. Soft-tissue abscesses should be incised and drained and antibiotic therapy instituted where appropriate.

Radicular Cyst

The radicular (periapical; dental) cyst is an inflammatory cyst arising from the epithelial residues in the periodontal membrane, usually following pulp necrosis. It is the most common cyst found in the jaws and develops when a pulp inflammation spreads to the periapical region to give rise to an apical granuloma. At this site, epithelial remnants proliferate, stimulated by inflammation, and result in an epithelial lined cystic cavity. Radicular cysts present radiographically as a well-defined radiolucency. The cyst lining comprises non-keratinized stratified squamous epithelium which may show mucoid metaplasia, cholesterol clefting and hyaline body formation. Surgical removal is the treatment of choice.

METABOLIC DISEASES OF THE JAWS

The three commonly occurring forms of generalized metabolic bone disease are osteoporosis, osteomalacia and osteitis fibrosa (the specific bone disease of hyperparathyroidism).

Osteoporosis

Osteoporosis is a disorder in which the bone is of normal composition but reduced in quantity. It represents a non-specific reaction of the skeleton to a number of different stimuli and constitutes one of the commonest of all bone disorders.

Osteoporosis is best considered as a normal ageing process in the skeleton of all adults, a process which may be further accelerated by, for example, immobilization, endocrine disease, or the administration of corticosteroids. However, in the majority of cases, a well-defined accelerating factor cannot be detected and in these circumstances the term 'idiopathic osteoporosis' is applied to the condition.

In most cases, the plasma levels of calcium, phosphorus and alkaline phosphatase are normal (Table 16.1). The level of faecal calcium is usually raised whilst urinary calcium excretion varies considerably, depending upon the stage of the disease.

Table 16.1. *Biochemical findings in metabolic bone disease.*

	Plasma				Urine
	Calcium	Phosphorus	Alkaline phosphatase	Urea	24-hr Calcium
Osteoporosis	N	N	N	N	N or ↑
Osteomalacia due to vitamin D deficiency or malabsorption	N or ↓	↓	↑	N	↓
Osteitis fibrosa 1μ or 3μ	↑	↓ or N or ↑	↑	N or ↑	↑ or N or ↓
2μ due to renal failure	N or ↓	N or ↓	↑	↑	↓
2μ due to vitamin D deficiency or malabsorption	N or ↓	↓	↑	N	↓
Paget's disease of bone	N	N	↑	N	N
Fibrous dysplasia	N	N	N or ↑	N	N

N = normal.

Osteoporosis is often asymptomatic, the diagnosis being made from radiographic evidence. Bone pain, especially in the lumbar region, is a common symptom whilst pathological fractures of the femoral neck may occur in the elderly. The jaw bones are affected as part of this generalized disease process.

The treatment of osteoporosis is complex. Any coexistent endocrine abnormality should be corrected. Exercise, together with analgesics, sex hormones, vitamin and mineral supplements, constitute the usual approach to arresting the disease process and alleviating the symptoms.

Rickets and Osteomalacia

Deficiency of vitamin D or resistance to its actions gives rise to rickets and osteomalacia. The effects are most profound in childhood and consist of localized swellings at epiphyseal plates and bowing of long bones (rickets). In adults, in whom the epiphyses are fused, the long bones are softened, resulting in bone pain, tenderness deformity or pathological fractures.

Diagnostic features include biochemical findings of low plasma calcium and phosphorus and raised alkaline phosphatase (Table 16.1) levels and, histologically, abnormally large amounts of osteoid.

Clinically, severe or prolonged vitamin D deficiency in childhood is not necessarily associated with dental changes. Thus, hypoplasia, delayed eruption or jaw bone changes are not features of the condition.

Hyperparathyroidism

The aetiology of this condition is usually a primary tumour of a gland or hyperplasia of one or more glands. Renal disease and steatorrhoea may cause a secondary form of hyperparathyroidism.

Primary hyperparathyroidism, caused by a parathyroid tumour's giving rise to hypercalcaemia and osteitis fibrosa, is distinguished from secondary hyperparathyroidism where excess hormone is produced as a compensatory reaction to prolonged renal—glomerular failure. The term 'tertiary hyperparathyroidism' is used to describe cases in which parathyroid tumours develop as a consequence of prolonged secondary hyperparathyroidism.

Clinical. The clinical picture is that of skeletal change, urinary abnormalities and serum calcium metabolic upset. Dull aches and pain occur in bones which later may exhibit deformity and even pathological fracture. Clubbing of fingers and toes may be observed. Urinary changes are those of high calcium output (2.5 mmol/l/24 hrs) (10 mg/100 ml/24 hrs) and high phosphate excretion (Table 16.1). The development of renal stones is common and renal failure may ensue. The tumour, usually an adenoma, often occurs in the inferior glands which are extremely difficult to palpate.

It is generally agreed that parathyroid hormone's (PTH) principal function is to maintain normal plasma calcium levels and that hypocalcaemia stimulates the secretion of PTH by a feedback mechanism. Direct action of PTH on bone leads to osteoclastic resorption, osteocytic osteolysis and varied osteoblastic activity. These actions account for the varied histological picture observed in the three types of hyperparathyroidism.

Pathology. The characteristic histopathological feature of osteitis fibrosa is osteoclastic resorption of bony trabeculae with fibrous replacement of the resorbed bone. Bone formation increases, with deposition of osteoid on bone surfaces. Brown-coloured soft-tissue masses may be formed, composed of osteoclast-like cells lying in spindle cell stroma which is highly vascular.

The osteoclastic resorption takes place as a consequence of parathormone stimulation. In the jaws, the typical histological features occur and cyst formation, 'brown tumours' containing giant cells, subperiosteal erosions and bone loss are observed. The giant cell lesions of hyperparathyroidism are indistinguishable histologically from the giant cell granuloma, whether central or peripheral. Clearly, hyperparathyroidism must be excluded in all cases of oral giant cell lesions.

Radiology. A radiolucent 'moth-eaten' appearance (Figure 16.3) is usual. Multiple cyst-like lesions may also be present. The lamina dura is reduced in thickness or absent and this may be an important diagnostic sign.

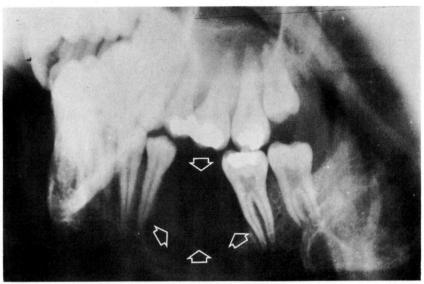

Figure 16.3. Radiographic appearance of the lesion of hyperparathyroidism affecting the mandible.

Diagnosis. The diagnosis is suggested by the clinical history and confirmed by the characteristic, radiological and biochemical features.

Treatment. Surgical treatment of primary and tertiary hyperparathyroidism has a good prognosis.

Acromegaly

An adenoma of the eosinophil cells of the anterior lobe of the pituitary gland, developing after epiphyseal closure, gives rise to acromegaly. Bones increase in thickness due to surface deposition, whilst subcutaneous tissue is also affected. Facial skin has a coarse appearance and the tongue and lips are thickened. Mandibular protrusion and overgrowth of the nasal cartilage produce a characteristic facial appearance. The hands and feet are enlarged, and severe headaches, voice deepening and diabetes insipidus are other clinical features of the condition.

Treatment. Approaches to treatment include surgical removal of the tumour, or radiotherapy.

FIBRO-OSSEOUS LESIONS

The term 'fibro-osseous' is often applied to lesions of the jaws with little regard to the criteria which should be adopted when considering the inclusion of a disease or lesion in this category. The term is best regarded as descriptive of the histology of certain diseases. It does not indicate any particular aetiology or nature of disease and may be applied as readily to certain disturbances of growth and maturation (dystrophies), as to some tumours and tumour-like swellings of unknown aetiology in bone. In the present chapter, fibrous dysplasia and Paget's disease of bone are included under the heading 'fibro-osseous lesions', and other lesions, which are also fibro-osseous in character, appear under other headings.

Fibrous Dysplasia of Bone

Although its aetiology is unknown, this disease is best considered as a disorder of development. The condition is characterized by the replacement of bone by fibrous tissue which may undergo metaplasia to form calcified tissue. With maturation of the skeleton the lesions tend to be self-limiting. Clinically, two types of fibrous dysplasia exist: polyostotic, where many bones are affected, and monostotic, where a single bone is affected. Polyostotic fibrous dysplasia frequently occurs in several bones of one limb, especially in the lower limbs. The monostotic type usually affects a limb, rib or jaw bone. The maxilla is affected more often than the mandible.

Clinical. The polyostotic form is usually seen in children. Skeletal deformities and pathological fractures, due to weakening as a result of bone replacement by fibrous and fibro-osseous tissue, may be observed. In the jaws, in the monostotic type, symptoms may be slight, the usual pattern being a gradually increasing facial asymmetry (Figure 16.4). On occasion, however, swelling may be rapid and extensive, giving rise to ocular and nasal symptoms.

Pain is not a feature of jaw involvement but dental abnormalities such as tooth displacement, occlusal abnormality and delayed eruption may arise. On palpation the lesions are bony-hard and non-tender. Biochemical investigations will occasionally reveal a raised serum alkaline phosphatase.

Radiology. Expansion of bone by cyst-like areas which have a mottled or opaque appearance, and which are caused by the metaplastic bone formation, is the usual pattern.

Pathology. Excised tissue is yellowish or grey-white in colour and is gritty on cutting. On occasion, multi-centric lesions may be present and, in addition, cystic spaces containing clear fluid or blood may be noted.

Histology. Normal bone is replaced by fibrous tissue in which osseous metaplasia occurs. The proportion of fibrous tissue decreases as the lesion matures. The fibrous tissue may be richly cellular with whorling of spindle cells. Alternatively, thick interlacing strands of collagen with a relative paucity of cells may dominate the histological picture. Bony trabeculae, irregular in size and shape, are most abundant in areas of cellular fibrous tissue. At first these comprise osteoid which later calcifies, and osteoblastic activity may be noted at their margins. Occasionally, osteoclastic activity is observed and giant cells may be noted at the edge of a lesion. Focal degeneration of fibrous tissue gives rise to micro- and macro-cyst formation together with the appearance of foamy macrophages.

Behaviour. The lesions tend to stabilize as the skeleton matures, but phases of renewed growth are not uncommon, especially during pregnancy.

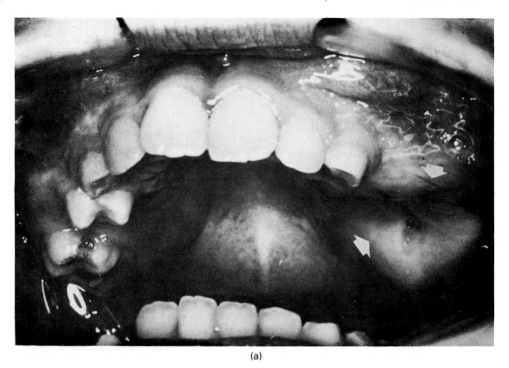

(a)

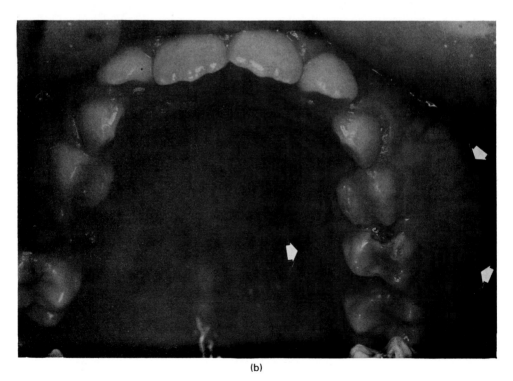

(b)

Figure 16.4. Palatal and buccal expansion of maxillary alveoli in fibrous dysplasia.

Treatment. Surgery should be deferred until skeletal growth ceases after puberty. Bone contouring may be required for cosmetic reasons at this stage. Radiotherapy is contra-indicated in view of the risk of neoplastic change and the problems caused by the effects of radiation on the facial tissues and the salivary glands.

Albright's Syndrome

This condition is usually observed in children and comprises the triad of polyostotic fibrous dysplasia with a tendency towards unilateral distribution; abnormal pigmentation of skin (Figure 16.5) and mucous membranes; and sexual precocity, especially in females, due to endocrine dysfunction. Other endocrinopathies, including hyperthyroidism, acromegaly and Cushing's disease, have been reported in association with the syndrome. The fundamental lesion may be a congenital hypothalamic abnormality causing over-production of a variety of hormones.

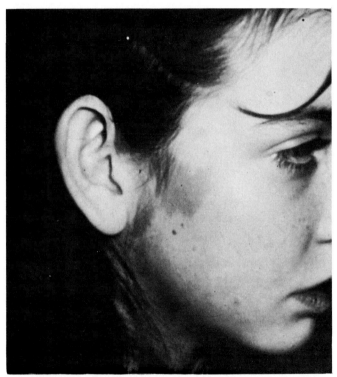

Figure 16.5. Skin pigmentation in a case of Albright's syndrome.

Paget's Disease of Bone

This condition, first described in 1887 by Sir James Paget, is a chronic bone dystrophy of unknown aetiology.

Striking geographical differences in incidence appear to exist. The condition is fairly common in the United Kingdom, France and Germany but comparatively rare in Scandinavia, central and southern Europe. The sex distribution is equal and the condition is essentially a disease of old age. Autopsy studies of unselected subjects have revealed an incidence of approximately 3 per cent among those who are over 40 years of age. Sporadic reports in families suggest the presence of a genetic factor, but this remains unidentified at the present time.

Clinical. Aching pain in affected bones, together with stiffness of joints, muscle weakness and fatigue, are common. Dilation of blood vessels gives rise to an increased skin temperature. The vertebrae are commonly involved, especially in the lumbar and sacral regions, indicating the existence of a stress factor. The skull, too, is commonly affected and the maxilla is a more frequent site than the mandible.

The classical polyostotic form of Paget's disease gives rise to progressive enlargement of the head, and a loss of height which is associated with kyphosis, enlargement and bowing of the bones of the lower limbs. In the head and neck an early symptom may be intermittent pain of the neuralgic type which may be severe. Bone enlargement leads to facial deformity whilst alveolar bone expansion leads to spacing of teeth and denture problems, together with temporomandibular dysfunction. Osteosarcoma may complicate Paget's disease of bone in 5 to 10 per cent of cases.

Pathology. Paget's disease reflects a combination of bone resorption and deposition occurring without relation to normal states and dynamics of the affected bone. The earliest change occurs in the haversian canals and consists of osteoclastic resorption. Adjacent resorbed spaces coalesce, exposing connective tissue marrow cells from which new bone is laid down as thin trabeculae. Continual resorption of old bone and deposition of new bone results in extensive remodelling, the tissue having an irregular mosaic pattern. Fluorescent isotope marker studies demonstrate a tenfold increase in the rate of bone turnover. New bone may form as small, acellular spheroidal masses that gradually enlarge and fuse, creating large areas of dense sclerotic bone. Hypercementosis of the teeth occurs after bony changes in the jaws are well established. The excessive cementum may be deposited in the same fashion as abnormal bone, with successive irregular increments and resorptions. In some cases, the net effect may be extensive root resorption. Fusion between dense bone and hyperplastic cementum may give rise to ankylosis. Clearly, the extraction of teeth will be complicated by the presence of hypercementosis (Figure 16.6) and ankylosis. Severe infection, too, may follow operative procedures to these dense avascular areas of bone formed in the osteosclerotic phase of the disease.

Radiology. Initially, a radiolucency is noted in affected bones and this is followed by a granular appearance. Thickening of the outer table of the skull with loss of distinction between diploë and irregular areas of sclerosis, giving rise to the 'cotton-wool' appearance, are also noted (Figure 16.7).

Biochemistry. Serum alkaline phosphatase is markedly increased in the active phase of the disease and may afford a measure of activity during the osteoclastic phase. The exact role of alkaline phosphatase is disputed but it is thought that the inhibitor of mineralization, inorganic pyrophosphate, is removed as a result of enzyme action. Thus, collagen of the matrix initiates crystallization of hydroxyapatite. When bone collagen is broken down during the resorptive phase, released hydroxyproline is not re-used and is either metabolized or excreted in the urine. The normal urinary daily excretion is 0.30 mmol (40 mg). In Paget's disease the rate may be 0.76 mmol/24 hrs (1 g/24 hrs).

Treatment. An advance in treatment has been the use of calcitonin. Calcitonin is a polypeptide (4000 mol. wt) produced by the C-cells of the thyroid. Its action is opposite to that of parathormone in that bone resorption is suppressed and there is a fall in blood calcium and phosphorus levels and also urinary hydroxyproline excretion. Synthetic human or porcine calcitonin may be used. It is given parenterally one to two times per day. Serum biochemical levels return to normal in several weeks and symptoms often dramatically improve. Bone histology returns to normal.

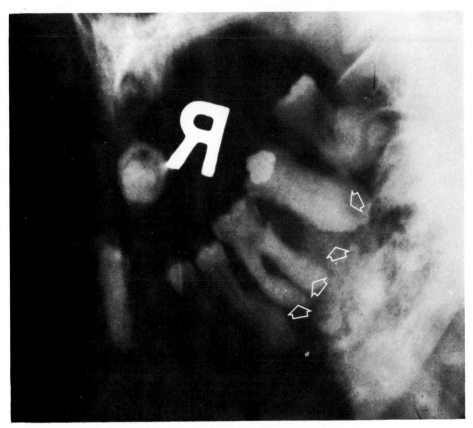

Figure 16.6. Cemental hyperplasia in Paget's disease of bone.

TUMOURS AND TUMOUR-LIKE SWELLINGS OF BONE

Solitary Bone Cyst

This unicameral cavity may present in the jaw bones of young and adolescent patients. The cavity is lined by a connective tissue membrane which is vascular and may show giant cells and cholesterol clefting. Pathological fracture may be a complication. The aetiology is unknown.

Aneurysmal Bone Cyst

These lesions are usually seen in patients under 30 years of age. They often have an eccentric location which, together with the 'ballooning-out' distension of the periosteum, is responsible for their name. The lesion is benign but its expansion may be rapid. Histologically, this expanding osteolytic lesion is characterized by blood-filled spaces with septa comprising connective tissue and bony trabeculae. Osteoid and giant cells are usually present.

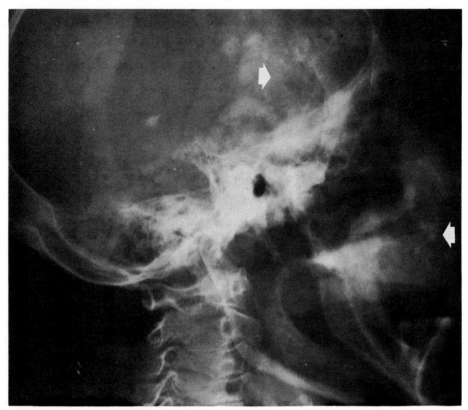

Figure 16.7. Loss of distinction between diploë and irregular areas of sclerosis in Paget's disease of bone.

Torus Palatinus and Mandibularis

These swellings represent non-neoplastic bony overgrowths. The torus palatinus is a bony overgrowth of the palatine process of the maxilla. Lesions of both palate and mandible appear at puberty and progress slowly thereafter. They may be removed for functional or prosthetic reasons, and do not recur.

Central Giant Cell Granuloma

This lesion of unknown aetiology is considered to represent a dysplasia of the resorptive tissue of bone: it is not a neoplasm. The lesion is associated with the tooth-bearing regions of the jaws and histologically shows loss of bone and replacement by plump fibroblasts and giant cells. Histologically, the picture is indistinguishable from the brown 'tumours' of hyperparathyroidism, and diagnosis of the latter must be excluded by appropriate investigations. Radiographically, a multilocular radiolucency may be noted. The lesion grows slowly but insidiously. Excision is curative.

Osteoma

This benign neoplasm may occur singly or may be multiple. It is confined to membrane bones and presents as a round well-defined hard swelling. Histologically, fine trabeculae of lamellar bone with intervening fatty or fibrous tissue are noted and the lesion is fundamentally that of dense bone. Occasionally, the tumour is subperiosteal and the attachment may be pedunculated. Recurrence after removal is not a feature of osteomas.

Osteomatosis

These are rare, multiple bone tumours that may affect maxilla and mandible. Clinically, small firm bony tumours may present in the palate and gingiva. Such lesions may occur in Gardner's syndrome, a familial condition of multiple bony tumours, cutaneous fibromas, epidermal cysts and polyposis coli. See Chapter 11 for more details.

Ossifying Fibroma

This is a central tumour which may be confused with fibrous dysplasia and is considered by some as a fibro-osseous lesion. It occurs at any age and in either jaw. The tumour is asymptomatic until it causes swelling or displacement of teeth. It consists of irregular ossification in a spindle cell stroma, the amount of ossification depending on the maturity of the lesion. The tumour should be removed surgically. Recurrence is uncommon.

Osteosarcoma

This is a relatively rare tumour, but amongst primary malignant lesions of bone it is the most common. It occurs less commonly in the jaws than in other bones.

Clinical. The tumour tends to occur in persons between 10 and 30 years of age and in the mandible rather than the maxilla. It presents as a rapidly growing tumour with swelling, pain, anaesthesia of the lip, loosening of teeth, and nasal obstruction and/or eye displacement, depending on the site of involvement.

Radiology. In the sclerotic type of lesion much bone is formed which gives a radiating 'sun-ray' appearance due to the formation of fine lamina at the periphery of the lesion. In the osteolytic type, the appearance is that of an irregular radiolucency. A combination of these two patterns is often noted.

Histology. The cardinal feature is the formation of neoplastic bone by malignant osteoblasts. These cells are pleomorphic and display malignant cytological characteristics. Abnormal mitosis may be present. The serum alkaline phosphatase level may be increased.

Relationship to pre-existing bone disease. Osteosarcoma may complicate Paget's disease in approximately 5 to 10 per cent of cases, whilst irradiation of the jaws may likewise induce malignant bone disease.

Behaviour and prognosis. This is a highly malignant tumour which shows early metastasis to the lungs.

Multiple Myeloma

Multiple myeloma is a malignant neoplasm of plasma cells and usually arises in the marrow, especially in the skull, vertebrae, ribs, sternum and pelvic bones. Myelomatous lesions account for 3 per cent of all bone tumours. Both multiple and solitary lesions occur in the jaws. The plasmacytoma is a soft-tissue lesion which may occur in lymph nodes, liver, spleen, other internal organs and also in the oral tissues.

Clinical. Myelomatosis occurs in middle-aged and elderly persons and males are affected about four times as frequently as females. The most frequent site of involvement is the skull in which there are lesions in over 70 per cent of cases. In about 30 per cent of cases, lesions of the jaws may be present and the mandible is much more commonly affected than the maxilla. In the jaws, pain is a common early symptom. Numbness of the lip, due to nerve involvement, loosening of teeth, pathological fractures and severe post-extraction haemorrhage, may be present. Swelling and tenderness are features and when the cortical plate is perforated the lesion appears as a soft-tissue fleshy mass.

Amyloidosis may accompany the condition and the tongue may be affected, its enlargement giving rise to problems of speech, mastication and swallowing. Patients with multiple myeloma are highly susceptible to infection which is induced by the impaired immune system. Anaemia frequently develops as a result of impairment of bone-marrow function. Multiple myeloma is rapidly fatal; duration is not longer than three to four years.

Radiology. Radiographic investigation reveals characteristic punched-out areas of rarefaction, frequently found in the skull and mandible. In the oral cavity, the lamina dura becomes less distinct and root resorption may occur in 10 per cent of patients.

Biochemical. Characteristic changes include alteration in serum protein distribution, Bence Jones proteinuria, elevated serum calcium level, excess of plasma cells in marrow puncture films, and anaemia.

Pathology. The lesion comprises a mass of tumour cells resembling inflammatory plasma cells but being slightly larger and showing binucleate forms. Mitosis may be present, and an occasional giant cell noted. The stroma is scanty.

Treatment. Urethan, cyclophosphamide and L-phenylalanine mustard have been employed in the treatment of multiple myeloma. All, however, give rise to serious side-effects which may take the form of marrow depression leading to leucopenia, anaemia and thrombocytopenia. These drugs prolong the course of the illness in some cases but the final outcome cannot be in doubt.

Solitary Myeloma

In a small number of cases, there occurs a single lesion of the jaws similar, histologically, to the lesion of multiple myeloma. Biochemical changes are absent. Such solitary myelomas may regress after surgical treatment but often further lesions appear and the disease is then recognized as multiple myeloma.

Metastatic Tumours in Bone

Primary carcinomas of bronchus, breast, prostate, kidney, thyroid and of other organs may disseminate via the blood stream to be deposited in the jaw bones.

Eosinophilic Granuloma

The eosinophilic granuloma is not a tumour. It, and similar lesions, occur in either solitary or multiple form, the latter as part of the Hand—Schüller—Christian syndrome or Letterer—Siwe disease. These conditions are often regarded as 'histiocytosis' or 'reticuloendotheliosis'. The young are affected and common sites of involvement are the skull, mandible, ribs, femur and flat bones. The lesions are osteolytic and may induce a periosteal reaction. Histologically, the eosinophilic granuloma is characterized by intense proliferation of reticulohistiocytic elements together with eosinophilic leucocytes, lymphocytes, plasma cells and giant cells. See Chapter 23.

TUMOURS OF ODONTOGENIC ORIGIN

Tumours arising from odontogenic epithelium usually occur in the jaws and require differentiation from many of the lesions discussed previously in this chapter. The recent classification by the World Health Organization is shown in Table 16.2.

Ameloblastoma

Ameloblastoma comprises approximately 1 per cent of all oral tumours. It has an equal sex distribution and the age range of patients is 20 to 50 years. The ameloblastoma is a benign but locally invasive neoplasm. Approximately 80 per cent of the lesions occur in the mandible, the majority being intra-osseous growths arising from odontogenic epithelium. However, a small proportion may arise from residues of epithelium lying outside bone. A few may arise as the result of neoplastic change within the wall of a non-neoplastic odontogenic cyst.

Clinical features. The lesion is slow growing, usually painless, with little displacement of teeth or obvious swelling in the initial stage.

Radiography. Usually a multilocular radiolucency is present although unilocular lesions occur. Considerable radiographic variation is the rule and the lesion requires differentiation from other cystic lesions. An embedded tooth may be present.

Pathology. The tumour consists of cords or columns or small rounded islands of epithelium lying in a fibrous tissue stroma. The peripheral epithelial cells are cuboidal or columnar in type and resemble pre-ameloblasts. The central cells are polyhedral and are similar to those of the stellate reticulum. Cyst formation is common. The connective tissue stroma is unremarkable. The histopathological pattern varies greatly. Follicular, plexiform, acanthomatous (showing squamous metaplasia), basal cell and granular cell types are described. These variations have little pathogenetic significance.

Behaviour. The tumour grows slowly but if left untreated will cause gross destruction of bone. On rare occasions, a true metastasis occurs.

Table 16.2. *Histological typing of odontogenic tumours, jaw cysts, and allied lesions.*

I. Neoplasms and other tumours related to the odontogenic apparatus

  A. Benign
1. Ameloblastoma
2. Calcifying epithelial odontogenic tumour
3. Ameloblastic fibroma
4. Adenomatoid odontogenic tumour (adeno-ameloblastoma)
5. Calcifying odontogenic cyst
6. Dentinoma
7. Ameloblastic fibro-odontoma
8. Odonto-ameloblastoma
9. Complex odontoma
10. Compound odontoma
11. Fibroma (odontogenic fibroma)
12. Myxoma (myxofibroma)
13. Cementomas
   (a) Benign cementoblastoma (true cementoma)
   (b) Cementifying fibroma
   (c) Periapical cemental dysplasia (periapical fibrous dysplasia)
   (d) Gigantiform cementoma (familial multiple cementomas)
14. Melanotic neuro-ectodermal tumour of infancy (melanotic progonoma; melano-ameloblastoma)

  B. Malignant
1. Odontogenic carcinomas
   (a) Malignant ameloblastoma
   (b) Primary intra-osseous carcinoma
   (c) Other carcinomas arising from odontogenic epithelium, including those arising from odontogenic cysts
2. Odontogenic sarcomas
   (a) Ameloblastic fibrosarcoma (ameloblastic sarcoma)
   (b) Ameloblastic odontosarcoma

II. Neoplasms and other tumours related to bone

  A. Osteogenic neoplasms
1. Ossifying fibroma (fibro-osteoma)

  B. Non-neoplastic bone lesions
1. Fibrous dysplasia
2. Cherubism
3. Central giant cell granuloma (giant cell reparative granuloma)
4. Aneurysmal bone cyst
5. Simple bone cyst (traumatic, haemorrhagic bone cyst)

III. Epithelial cysts

  A. Developmental
1. Odontogenic
   (a) Primordial cyst (keratocyst)
   (b) Gingival cyst
   (c) Eruption cyst
   (d) Dentigerous (follicular) cyst
2. Non-odontogenic
   (a) Nasopalatine duct (incisive canal) cyst
   (b) Globulomaxillary cyst
   (c) Nasolabial (naso-alveolar) cyst

  B. Inflammatory
1. Radicular cyst

IV. Unclassified lesions

From WHO.

Treatment is by surgical excision.

Calcifying Epithelial Odontogenic Tumour

This tumour, also called Pindborg's tumour, is a locally invasive epithelial neoplasm characterized by the development of intra-epithelial structures, probably amyloid in nature. Portions of the lesion may calcify.

Clinical. There is an equal sex distribution with an age range of 20 to 60 years. The mandible is affected more commonly than the maxilla, especially in the premolar/molar region. The majority of lesions are associated with the coronal aspect of an unerupted tooth. A few are not associated with teeth whilst rarely the lesion may be present in an extra-osseous location.

Radiology. The usual radiographic appearance is an irregular radiolucent area containing radio-opaque masses of varying size.

Histology. Within a connective tissue stroma, polyhedral epithelial cells with prominent intercellular bridges are observed. Mitoses are rare, although the epithelial cells may be multinuclear and show pleomorphism. Rounded, acidophilic homogeneous masses which calcify and give positive reactions for amyloid are noted. The epithelial cells commonly degenerate, thus liberating these masses. The lesion is judged to arise from remnants of the reduced enamel epithelium.

Treatment. The lesion is locally invasive but complete resection is curative. Curettage may be followed by recurrence.

Ameloblastic Fibroma

This neoplasm comprises proliferating odontogenic epithelium within a cellular mesodermal tissue which resembles dental papilla. However, odontoblasts are not formed.

Clinical. Young patients around 20 years of age are most commonly affected. The mandibular molar/premolar region is the site of predilection. The lesion grows slowly and painlessly.

Radiology. A well-defined radiolucency characterizes the radiographic appearance.

Histology. The lesion tends to be encapsulated and has the appearance of a soft firboma. Epithelial strands, or islands, which have a peripheral cuboidal layer enclosing stellate reticulum-like regions are noted. A highly cellular connective tissue stroma is present. A narrow cell-free zone may border the epithelium although this may represent a fixation artefact.

Treatment. The lesion is benign and should be excised.

Adenomatoid Odontogenic Tumour

This tumour of odontogenic epithelium forms duct-like structures and exhibits varying degrees of inductive change within the supporting connective tissue stroma.

Clinical. The sex distribution is equal and the lesion generally presents in the second decade. The tumour is slow-growing, usually painless and affects the maxilla, especially in the canine region, more than the mandible.

Radiology. The radiographic features are those of a well-circumscribed radiolucency with occasional radiopacities. The lesion is often associated with an unerupted tooth.

Histology. The lesion tends to be cystic in nature. The epithelial tumour cells form strands, sheets and whorled masses, the over-all pattern having a duct-like appearance. The nuclei are polarized away from the central space which contains homogeneous PAS-positive eosinophilic material. The connective tissue stroma tends to show hyalinization, often with strands of entrapped epithelium. This may represent dysplastic dentine.

Treatment. The lesion is readily enucleated and does not recur.

Calcifying Odontogenic Cyst

The lesion presents in a fashion similar to that of a developmental cyst of the jaws. Radiographically, there is a well-defined radiolucency with varying amounts of radio-opaque material. The lesion occurs within bone but occasionally may arise in soft tissues of tooth-bearing areas.

Histology. The cyst lining shows a well-defined basal layer of columnar cells and an overlying layer reminiscent of stellate reticulum. Amorphous 'ghost' cells are noted, and these often calcify. Dysplastic dentine may be formed adjacent to the basal layer of epithelium.

Treatment. Recurrence is most uncommon and enucleation is usually curative.

Complex Odontoma

This is a malformation in which all dental tissues are represented. All tissues are well formed but they occur in a fairly disorganized manner. The mandible is the most common site.

Compound Odontoma

In this malformation, the dental tissues are represented in a more orderly fashion, producing tooth-like masses.

Odontogenic Fibroma

This is a fibroblastic neoplasm containing variable amounts of odontogenic epithelium. This fibrous tissue is mature whilst the epithelial component is scanty.

Odontogenic Myxoma

This locally invasive neoplasm consists of clumps of rounded epithelial cells in an abundant myxomatous stroma. Radiographically, multiple radiolucent 'soap-bubble' areas are noted. There is little attempt at encapsulation and growth may be rapid.

Cementomas

These lesions containing cementum-like tissue form a complex group with ill-defined characteristics.

Benign Cementoblastoma

Sheets of cementum-like material are formed and reversal lines may be seen. Radiographically, a well-defined radio-opaque lesion with a peripheral radiolucent zone is noted. The lesion is associated with the root of a premolar or molar tooth, usually in the lower jaw. It is benign and readily enucleated.

Cementifying Fibroma

This tumour comprises cellular fibroblastic tissue which contains rounded, calcified masses of cementum-like tissue. It is usually noted in the mandible in older individuals.

Periapical Cemental Dysplasia

The tumour is similar, histologically, to the cementifying fibroma, but often involves several teeth. It is commonly observed in the mandibular incisor region in middle-aged females.

Gigantiform Cementoma

This appears as a mass of dense, highly-calcified cementum, occurring in several parts of the jaws.

FURTHER READING

Lucas, R. B. (1976) *Pathology of Tumours of the Oral Tissues,* 3rd ed. Edinburgh: Churchill Livingstone.
Kelley, H. C., Kay, L. W. & Seward, G. R. (1977) *Benign Cystic Lesions of the Jaws, their Diagnosis and Treatment,* 3rd ed. Edinburgh: Churchill Livingstone.
Mason, D. K. & Chisholm, D. M. (1975) *Salivary Glands in Health and Disease.* London, Philadelphia, Toronto: W. B. Saunders.
Pindborg, J. J. (1970) *Pathology of the Dental Hard Tissues.* Philadelphia, London, Toronto: W. B. Saunders.
Shafer, W. G., Hine, M. K. & Levy, B. M. (1974) *A Textbook of Oral Pathology,* 3rd ed. Philadelphia, London, Toronto: W. B. Saunders.

Connective Tissue Disease

INTRODUCTION

The connective tissue diseases comprise a group of disorders of unknown aetiology, classified together because of the similarity of the tissue changes which occur in them. These changes are in no way specific for the connective tissues but merely represent the limited number of ways in which connective tissue may respond to injury. The connective tissue diseases include systemic lupus erythematosus, rheumatoid arthritis, systemic sclerosis, polyarteritis nodosa and dermatomyositis. There is good evidence for an autoimmune basis to these diseases which often occur together in one individual. The term 'connective tissue disease' stresses the principal site of involvement whilst 'autoimmune' refers to a pathogenic mechanism.

The problem of aetiology and pathogenesis of the connective tissue diseases is far from solved. In all probability the causation is multifactorial, with genetic, infective, immunological and environmental components playing a part.

RHEUMATOID ARTHRITIS

Rheumatoid arthritis is a slowly progressive, chronic, inflammatory disease of connective tissue which affects joints and may lead to permanent deformity. The condition is described more fully in Chapter 18.

Females are affected three times more frequently than males and the usual age of onset is in the third or fourth decade. The onset may be abrupt or insidious and at first the smaller diarthrodial joints are affected. Increasing destruction of the articular cartilages may lead to fibrous ankylosis and permanent deformity.

Oral Manifestations

The temporomandibular joint is affected in 10 to 15 per cent of cases, and pain, swelling and limitation of movement are the usual clinical features. Oral dryness (Figure 17.1) and salivary gland swelling are the hallmarks of Sjögren's syndrome (Chapter 14) in which rheumatoid arthritis is the common connective tissue disorder accompanying the condition.

Treatment

A glycerine and lemon mouthwash may alleviate oral dryness whilst general measures include rest, nutrition, drug therapy, physiotherapy and surgical correction of deformities. Among the anti-rheumatic drugs are salicylates, gold compounds, phenylbutazone, indomethacin and corticosteroids. Reactions to these drugs may result in oral lesions.

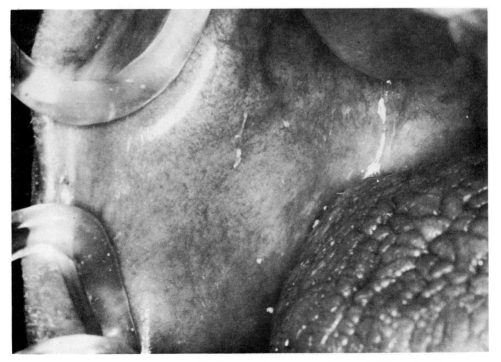

Figure 17.1. Severe oral dryness and 'pebble-stone' appearance of tongue in Sjögren's syndrome.

SYSTEMIC LUPUS ERYTHEMATOSUS

General

This is a serious constitutional disorder of unknown aetiology having protean manifestations. It may affect skin, mucosae, blood vessels, brain, heart, kidneys and white cells. Young females between the ages of 10 and 40 are particularly prone to develop the disease, whilst approximately 85 per cent of cases of any age are female. The course of the disease is varied and may extend over a period of years.

It is important to distinguish between the two forms of lupus erythematosus; systemic and cutaneous. These variations, however, are best considered as reflecting a spectrum of change. Cutaneous lupus erythematosus or chronic discoid lupus erythematosus is a chronic and recurrent disorder. A sharply circumscribed macular rash of skin and, on occasion, the oral mucosa characterizes the condition. The cause is unknown, although exposure to sunlight frequently precedes the initial appearance of the lesions and often causes exacerbation of them. Treatment is usually by topical steroid, but anti-malarial drugs such as hydroxychloroquine, given orally, may be of value.

Systemic lupus erythematosus gives rise to cutaneous lesions, the characteristic malar 'butterfly' rash (Figure 17.2) being only one of several erythematosus skin rashes which may occur. Articular, pulmonary, cardiac and renal symptoms, together with central nervous system involvement producing epilepsy and psychoses, may be noted.

Fibrinoid necrosis and bodies of altered nuclear material — 'haematoxylin bodies' — may be found in affected tissues. Antinuclear antibodies with the L.E. cell factor are

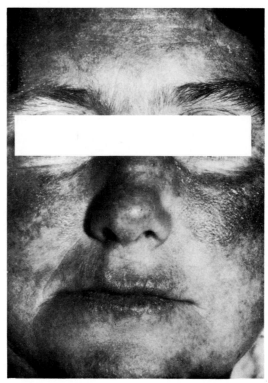

Figure 17.2. 'Butterfly' rash in a patient with lupus erythematosus.

present in the serum of most patients. The presence of antinuclear factor and DNA antibodies is an important diagnostic parameter. Anaemia, leucopenia and thrombocytopenia may be severe. Multiple serum protein abnormalities may occur and immunoglobulins are generally elevated.

Oral Manifestations

The oral cavity may be affected in a number of ways in this multi-system disorder. Involvement of the salivary glands will give rise to Sjögren's syndrome (see Chapter 14) in 1 to 10 per cent of cases. In general, mucosal lesions occur in 10 to 20 per cent of patients with systemic lupus erythematosus and are thus a significant finding. Purpuric lesions such as ecchymoses and petechiae can occur and oral ulceration is a feature. In chronic discoid lupus erythematosus there may be keratotic scaling of the vermilion border of the lips and dark red erythematous areas with peripheral keratosis may affect the oral mucosa (Figures 17.3 and 17.4). Ulcerative mucosal lesions which develop may heal with fibrosis and scarring. Herpetic and candidal infections appear to be more common in systemic lupus erythematosus and the latter often occurs in discoid lupus.

Treatment

The treatment and prognosis depend upon the severity and extent of the disease. Salicylates, corticosteroids, anti-malarial drugs and antimetabolic alkylating agents may be used.

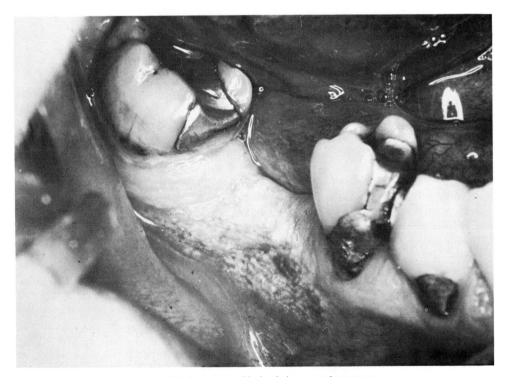

Figure 17.3. Oral mucosal lesion in lupus erythematosus.

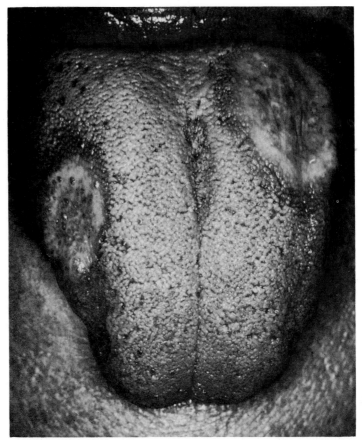

Figure 17.4. Lingual mucosal lesions in a patient with lupus erythematosus.

PROGRESSIVE SYSTEMIC SCLEROSIS

General

This is a chronic disease characterized by a diffuse sclerosis of the skin, gastrointestinal tract, heart, muscle, lungs and kidneys. Females between the ages of 20 and 50 are most commonly affected. The onset and course are usually insidious. Cutaneous changes include induration, hyperpigmentation and telangiectasia. Raynaud's phenomenon (digital arterial insufficiency provoked by cold) (Figure 17.5) is a common feature. Calcification of subcutaneous tissue is a late manifestation. Clinical symptoms will vary according to the extent and organ involvement of the disease. Thus cardiac, pulmonary, renal and gastrointestinal symptoms may be present. Hypergamma-globulinaemia and circulating serum autoantibodies are present in most cases.

A localized form of the disease, termed 'morphea' or 'localized scleroderma', is a benign self-limiting disease affecting the skin.

Histologically, in the early stages, collagen is oedematous and infiltrated by lymphocytes having a perivascular distribution. Later, collagen bundles become sclerotic and compressed. Elastic tissue is greatly diminished, skin appendages become atrophic and blood vessel walls show thickening with luminal narrowing.

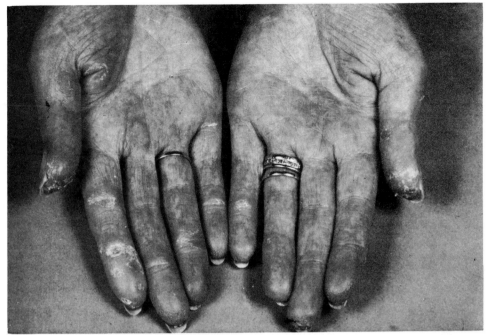

Figure 17.5. Raynaud's phenomenon, showing superficial necrosis of the skin. This phenomenon can occur in both systemic lupus erythematosus and progressive systemic sclerosis.

Orofacial Manifestations

When the face is involved, it becomes mask-like and expressionless (Figure 17.6). Involvement of lips and cheeks (Figures 17.7 and 17.8) make mastication and temporomandibular joint movement difficult: indeed, the temporomandibular joint may become fixed. Induration and immobility of the tongue interfere with mastication, swallowing and speech. The teeth may become protrusive and cause erosions of the immobile buccal and labial mucosa. Marked thickening of the periodontal membrane may be a prominent oral sign noted radiographically.

Treatment

Systemic steroids, physiotherapy and lubricative creams are employed in the therapy of this condition.

POLYARTERITIS NODOSA

General

This disease is characterized by segmental necrosis and inflammation of the walls of small- and medium-sized arteries, leading to the impairment of the blood supply to tissues served by the affected vessels. The course may be short or prolonged, and the manifestations are protean, being determined largely by the extent and sites of the lesions.

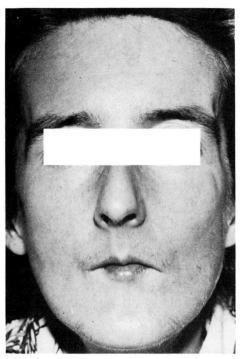

Figure 17.6. Mask-like appearance of scleroderma (systemic sclerosis).

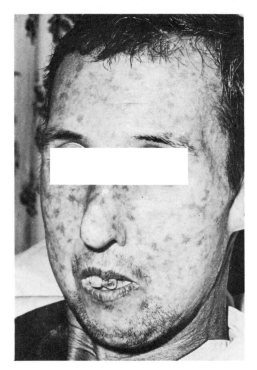

Figure 17.7. Sclerotic lesions of skin and microstomia in a patient with scleroderma.

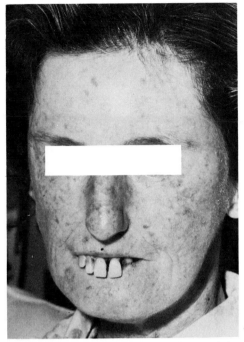

Figure 17.8. Involvement of skin and lips resulting in microstomia in scleroderma.

The histopathological features are segmental necrosis, fibrinoid degeneration and chronic inflammation. Any organ may be affected but the kidneys are the most commonly affected.

Oral Manifestations

Oral lesions are extremely rare, although oral ulceration has been reported. Purpuric lesions, similar to those in other connective tissue disorders, may also be seen. Patients may complain of muscle and joint pain, and peripheral nerve function may be disturbed.

The diagnosis depends largely upon biopsy. The disease is usually fatal though life may be prolonged by the use of corticosteroids.

DERMATOMYOSITIS

General

This is an inflammatory and degenerative disease of skin, muscles and, occasionally, of other organs. It may occur at any age but is most commonly found in middle life. Weakness and tenderness of the affected muscles, fever, skin eruptions (Figure 17.9) and progressive wasting are the characteristic features. The prognosis is poor and death usually results from respiratory or cardiac failure or from superimposed infection. An association with a malignant tumour in approximately 15 per cent of adult cases has been noted. Histologically, the muscles show focal necrosis and chronic inflammatory cell infiltration, often in the perimysium near blood vessels. The cutaneous lesions have no specific pattern, although an erythematous macular rash is described. Poikilo-dermatous change, with telangiectasis and atrophy, may develop during the later stages of the disease.

Oral Manifestations

The tongue may be affected in dermatomyositis, with a resultant tenderness, pain and weakness. During the early stage of the disease oedema may be a conspicuous feature, giving way, however, to atrophy as the disease progresses. Mucosal erosions of a non-specific type may be present in some cases.

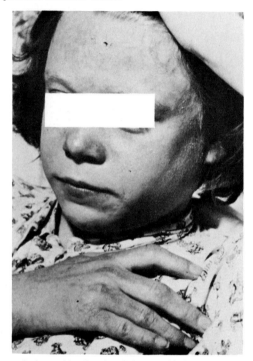

Figure 17.9. Cutaneous lesions of forehead and circumorbital region in a case of dermatomyositis.

Treatment

Systemic corticosteroids are the most useful therapy. The prognosis is variable and investigation for an underlying malignant tumour is indicated.

REITER'S SYNDROME

General

The triad of conjunctivitis, urethritis and arthritis constitutes Reiter's syndrome. It usually occurs in males who are 20 to 35 years of age, although isolated occurrences in females and children have been reported. Intensive efforts to establish a causative agent for this syndrome have failed. Among aetiological factors which have been suggested are venereal infection, mycoplasmal infection, bacillary dysentery and genetic and autoimmune mechanisms. Characteristic lesions include keratoderma blennorrhagicum, circinate balanitis, periostitis and oral ulceration.

Oral Manifestations

The main oral findings in Reiter's disease or syndrome are painless superficial erosions on the palate, buccal mucosa (Figure 17.10) and dorsum of the tongue. These red, glistening lesions progress to shallow erosions.

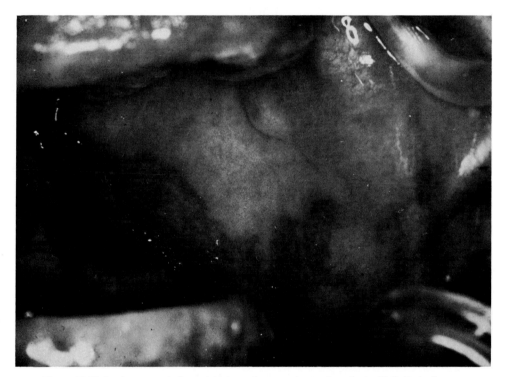

Figure 17.10. Erythematous lesions of the buccal mucosa in a male patient with Reiter's disease.

Treatment

Treatment is symptomatic. Bed rest, suitable diet, analgesics, and anti-inflammatory drugs, including steroids, have all been utilized in the management of this disorder.

OTHER CONNECTIVE TISSUE DISEASES WITH ORAL MANIFESTATIONS

The orofacial manifestations of rheumatoid arthritis (see Chapter 18), Sjögren's syndrome (see Chapter 14) and Behçet's syndrome (Chapter 3) are described elsewhere in the text. Paraproteinaemias may accompany connective tissue disease, and purpuric lesions, haemorrhagic diathesis and hyperviscosity syndrome with oral ulcers and bleeding may be present with macroglobulinaemia and cryoglobulinaemia.

Amyloidosis, as a secondary phenomenon in these chronic diseases, may affect the gingivae. Macroglossia caused by amyloid deposition is usually seen only in the primary form of the disease.

MUCOSAL REACTION TO DRUG THERAPY IN CONNECTIVE TISSUE DISEASE

Toxicity to gold, which is often used in the treatment of rheumatoid arthritis, is frequent, and dermatitis and stomatitis may occur. A metallic taste may accompany the stomatitis. Immunosuppressives and antimetabolite drugs may be toxic to bone marrow and may ultimately lead to mucosal and gingival haemorrhage. Folic acid antagonists may give rise to stomatitis and cheilitis. Secondary bacterial and fungal infection is common in the connective tissue diseases, partly as a consequence of drug therapy. The antimalarial drugs may cause oral pigmentation.

SUMMARY

The oral manifestations of some connective tissue diseases, for example Sjögren's syndrome, are features necessary to the establishment of the diagnosis. In other connective tissue diseases, oral involvement is frequent and significant, giving rise to problems in management. In many of the diseases, in contrast, the oral component is of little significance. Recognition of these lesions, together with knowledge of possible drug effects and the tendency to recurrent infection, are important parts of oral medicine.

FURTHER READING

Anderson, J. R., Buchanan, W. W. & Goudie, R. B. (1967) *Autoimmunity: Clinical and Experimental.* Illinois: Charles C. Thomas.
McCarthy, P. L. & Shklar, G. (1964) *Diseases of the Oral Mucosa.* New York: McGraw-Hill.

chapter 18

Temporomandibular Joint Disease

Introduction
Developmental Abnormalities
Trauma
Infections
Rheumatoid Arthritis
Osteoarthritis
Ankylosis
Facial Pain Dysfunction Syndrome

INTRODUCTION

General Considerations

In general, the temporomandibular joint is subject to those disorders which affect other articulations.

The most common disease of all joints, including the temporomandibular joint, is osteoarthritis. Rheumatoid arthritis is a less common disorder affecting the temporomandibular joint. Trauma resulting in fractures of the condyle leads to temporomandibular joint complications. Neoplastic disease affecting this joint is rare. In the practice of oral medicine, the facial pain dysfunction syndrome accounts for the greatest number of patients with temporomandibular joint symptoms. In general, problems involving this particular joint are mainly traumatogenic, pathogenic or psychogenic in origin.

Anatomical Considerations

There are several anatomical and functional characteristics of the temporomandibular joint articulation that set it apart from other joints. These may be listed as follows:

1. The joint is truly bilateral, the rigid mandibular connection between both joints preventing unilateral motion.

209

2. The articular surfaces are covered by avascular fibrous tissue, rather than by hyaline cartilage which is to be found in most joints.
3. The dentition acts as a guide or stop for joint movements.
4. A fibrous disc is situated between the temporal bone above and the condylar head below, thus dividing the joint into two compartments: an upper, which acts as a gliding joint and a lower, which acts as a hinge joint.

Functional Considerations

Functional and anatomical relationships exist among the dentition, the periodontal tissues, the muscles of mastication and the joint. This system may be regarded as a distinct physiological unit whose compartments are mutually dependent. A pathological condition in one compartment may affect the others.

The psychological implications of oral function are well documented and undoubtedly play a part in disease of this functional unit. Trauma to teeth and musculature may also affect joint movement. Thus, the joint is subject to the physiological and emotive functions of the oral cavity.

Radiology of the Temporomandibular Joint

Radiographic examination of the temporomandibular joint can be a demanding procedure. In practice, the amount of useful information gained by radiography is limited. In many cases, disturbances of joint movement are easily observed clinically as they are radiographically. Thus, the place of radiography is to detect overt joint disease. The technique of greatest value, in this respect, is the orthopantomograph (Figure 18.1). The short-distance transpharyngeal technique is of value where the bony structure of the condyle and condylar head are to be visualized (Figure 18.2). For the anterior—posterior view of the condylar head and neck, the transorbital anterior—posterior can be recommended, and tomography is often helpful. Clearly, radiographic investigation is of great value in cases of fractures of the condyle (Figure 18.3), dislocations (Figure 18.4) and neoplasms.

DEVELOPMENTAL ABNORMALITIES

Developmental abnormalities may be genetically determined or may result from prenatal or post-natal injury. Some are congenital, others develop during the years of growth. The abnormality present is usually reflected as hypoplasia, hyperplasia or agenesis of one or both condylar heads. Fortunately, these conditions are rare. They include the following:

Mandibulofacial Dysostosis

This is acquired as an autosomal dominant trait. Hypoplasia of condyle may be present and the degree is variable.

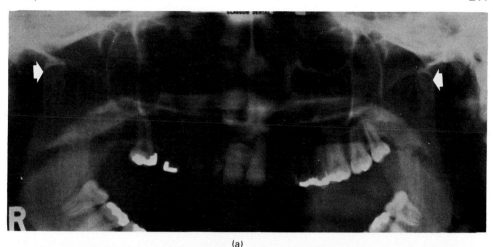

(a)

(b)

Figure 18.1. Orthopantomograph, showing normal temporomandibular joint relationships.

Developmental Condylar Agenesis

This is an extremely rare condition but may occur either unilaterally or bilaterally.

Hurler's Syndrome and Hunter's Syndrome

These disorders are grouped within the mucopolysaccharidoses or genetically determined disorders of carbohydrate metabolism.

Poor development of the condylar head may be present in some cases.

Unilateral Condylar Hyperplasia

The enlargement produces asymmetry and deviation of the jaw towards the unaffected side. A fairly typical malocclusion is usually present. Joint pain may also be present.

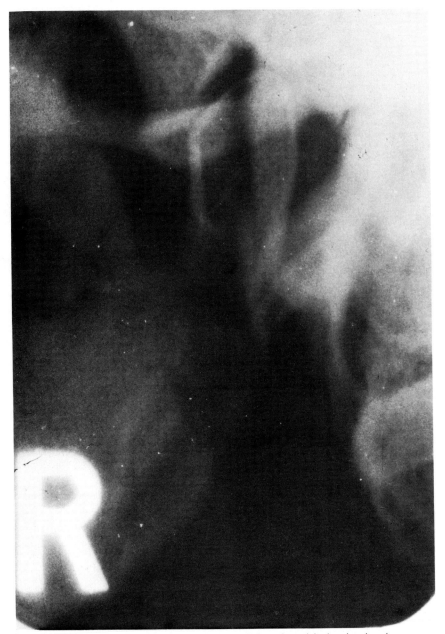

Figure 18.2. Short-distance transpharyngeal view of condylar head and neck.

Secondary Condylar Hypoplasia

This occurs when the head of the condyle is injured during development. Usually, trauma or infection can be implicated. If the injury is unilateral, deviation towards the affected side will produce the condition of cross-bite occlusion.

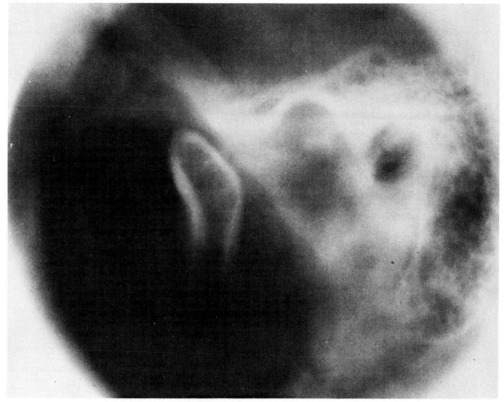

Figure 18.3. Condylar neck fracture.

TRAUMA

Acute Trauma

Acute trauma may lead to inflammatory reactions within the joint space (i.e. arthritis) or extravasation of blood into the joint (i.e. haemarthrosis). Further complications may be dislocation of the condyle or fracture of the condyle (especially a blow to the chin). From a diagnostic point of view, a history of trauma can usually be elicited. Pain, trismus, limitation of movement and deviation towards the injured side are also to be noted. Radiographs are required to exclude the possibility that fracture has occurred.

Subluxation

This refers to an incomplete or partial anterior dislocation of the condyle from the glenoid fossa. It implies that the condyle moves anteriorly over the articular eminence during opening. It is a hypermobility and the patient is able to self-reduce the subluxation. The clinical features are as follows:

1. Pain (especially in the last few mm of opening)
2. Clicking of the joint
3. Malocclusion of teeth

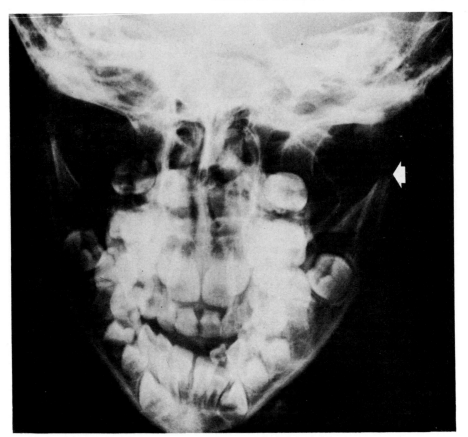

Figure 18.4. Anterior dislocation of the condyle.

Subluxation may follow, or it may be a complication of, the following:

1. Endotracheal intubation
2. Dental and oral treatment
3. Yawning
4. Osteoarthritis.

Dislocation (Luxation)

This refers to a non-self-reducing dislocation or displacement of the condyle from the glenoid fossa. The condyle may be displaced anteriorly, posteriorly or centrally (upward): anterior dislocation is the most common. The condyle is locked forward suddenly by spasm of temporal, internal pterygoid and/or masseter muscles. This results in protrusion of the mandible and open-bite. The chin is directed downwards and forward.

Pain, difficulty in eating, increased salivation and pre-auricular prominence are apparent.

If the dislocation is unilateral, there is a deviation towards the unaffected side. Some of the predisposing factors for dislocation are trauma, infection, degenerative changes and surgical operations (mouth props). Such physiological factors as the failure of the external pterygoid to relax in closing movements in those individuals whose condyles pass over the eminence, and myospasm of the masseter or the internal pterygoid muscles when these muscles are stretched by wide opening, thus pulling the condyle superiorly into the infratemporal fossa, may account for the condition.

INFECTIONS

Infections of the temporomandibular joint apparatus may occur as part of a systemic generalized infection, although this is a rare cause. A penetrating wound and the spread of infection from adjacent structures, such as the external ear canal, ramus of mandible or pterygoid fossa, are other causes.

Infections may be acute or chronic, systemic or local. The clinical features include pain, swelling and deformities. In addition, there is an increased susceptibility to later osteoarthritis and to adhesions which are either fibrous or bony.

Total loss of condyle due to osteomyelitis may occur and, in children, mal-development of the jaw due to disturbance of the mandibular growth centre is a serious complication.

RHEUMATOID ARTHRITIS

Rheumatoid arthritis is a slowly progressive, chronic inflammatory disease of connective tissue which affects joints and may lead to permanent deformity. It appears to be more common in those living in a temperate climate. The onset may be abrupt or insidious. At first there is an acute polysynovitis of the smaller diarthrodeal joints but, in time, the disease leads to increasing destruction of articular cartilage and to fibrous ankylosis. Females are affected three times more frequently than males. The usual age of onset is the third and fourth decade. Juvenile rheumatoid arthritis (Still's disease) has, of course, a much earlier age of onset. The aetiology is unknown, although bacterial and hormonal factors, heredity, immunological derangement and autoimmunity have been suggested as causal agents.

Rheumatoid arthritis is characterized by a chronic and progressive inflammation of joints, atrophy of muscles and rarefaction of bone.

The articular lesion in rheumatoid arthritis is a hypertrophic villous synovitis. Synovial tissue becomes thickened, a chronic inflammatory cell infiltrate is present and articular cartilage is replaced by granulation tissue. These destructive changes lead to loss of function and limitation of joint movement.

Involvement of temporomandibular joint is but a localized reflection of this systemic disease; it may, though rarely, be the first joint to become involved. Temporomandibular joint involvement in rheumatoid arthritis ranges from 10 per cent to more than 50 per cent of cases. This complication usually presents bilaterally and simultaneously.

Pain, swelling, tenderness, stiffness, crepitation and limitation of movement are the clinical features. Radiographs may show osteoporosis, limitation of movement, flattening of the condylar head and marginal surface irregularities.

Treatment includes rest, nutrition, drug therapy, physiotherapy and surgical correction of deformities. Included among the anti-rheumatic drugs are salicylates, gold compounds, phenylbutazone, indomethacin and corticosteroids.

OSTEOARTHRITIS

This is a degenerative, non-inflammatory joint disease which affects older individuals. Large, weightbearing joints are usually affected first. The lesions are characterized by deterioration and abrasion of articular surfaces and also by formation of new bone at the joint surfaces.

The disease has an insidious onset that is first noticed as a slight stiffness or decreased mobility in the affected joints. Faulty posture, obesity and occupational stress all predispose to the condition. There are no constitutional signs of an inflammatory disease. In some cases, however, the presence of Heberden's nodes about the bases of the terminal phalanges of the fingers may be noted. No laboratory findings of note exist. The erythrocyte sedimentation rate (ESR) may be raised and, radiographically, osteophytic formations may be observed. This latter feature results from destruction of hyaline cartilage followed by bone overgrowth.

Clinically, the temporomandibular joint may be affected in approximately 30 per cent of cases. Stiffness of the joint (especially when awakening) and clicking, usually in the absence of pain, are present. Chronic subluxation may occur but ankylosis is rare.

Radiographs, especially circular tomography, of the temporomandibular joint in affected cases show calcified shreds of articular tissue — osteophytes; small, subarticular radiolucencies — 'Ely's cysts'; areas of degeneration; flattening of condylar articular surface and posterior surface of eminence flattening.

Histologically the peripheral fibres of the surface fibrous articular layer loosen, with later denudation and eburnation of the bone end plate. Fibrosis occurs in the sub-articular marrow spaces and microfractures of the end plate and small cysts which form beneath it lead to its collapse and loss. Eventually a new end plate is formed and clinically normal function returns.

Treatment includes drug therapy with salicylates and indomethacin, and weight reduction. Surgical procedures, such as hip fusion or cup arthroplasty, may benefit some patients, and total hip replacement by metal prosthesis has an important role to play.

ANKYLOSIS (HYPOMOBILITY)

Immobility of the jaw may be

1. Uni- or bilateral
2. Intra- or extra-articular ('true or false')
3. Fibrous or bony
4. Partial or complete

Frequently, a combination of these occur in any one case.

Complete immobility is rare, even in bilateral bony ankylosis. An opening of 5 mm or less is considered sufficient to diagnose complete ankylosis. The condition is most frequently acquired, although it may be congenital. Intra-articular and unilateral ankyloses are the most common and, in this situation, deviation is towards the affected side. There is usually little pain or difficulty with speech. However, mastication is difficult and oral hygiene tends to be poor.

In children, the mandibular growth centre may be traumatized leading, ultimately, to severe disfigurement such as micrognathia and receding chin. The traumatic causes are varied but include birth injury (forceps delivery); trauma; infection; juvenile rheumatoid arthritis; trismus of muscles of mastication; and Paget's disease of bone. The treatment is surgical, but complications are common.

FACIAL PAIN DYSFUNCTION SYNDROME (TEMPOROMANDIBULAR JOINT SYNDROME)

Clinical

Facial pain dysfunction syndrome refers to a symptom complex of crepitation, decreased mobility, pre-auricular and auricular pain, pain on movement, headache, tenderness on palpation and, sometimes, nasopharyngeal symptoms.

It is clear, however, that the temporomandibular joint, the muscles of mastication and the dentition form a mutually interdependent system whereby organic derangement of one must affect the others. With regard to the age and sex distribution of the syndrome approximately 80 to 90 per cent of cases are female, and the majority are under 40 years of age. The most consistent symptoms are pain over the joints, which is elicited by pressure or movement, clicking during movement, which is usually unilateral, and deviation of the jaw, on opening, to the affected side. Radiographs are unhelpful in the majority of cases, whilst histopathological examination of material from the joint may show degenerative changes, though whether these are considered to be primary or secondary changes is dependent upon one's favoured aetiological concept.

The main aetiological considerations are over-closure of the mandible, occlusal abnormalities, internal derangement of joint, and spasm of the muscles of mastication together with generalized muscle tension. A psychosomatic factor operates in some cases.

The differences of opinion usually do not reflect clearly distinct mechanisms but tend, rather, to emphasize one or other of the components. Most commonly cases involve muscles of mastication and there is spasm of these muscles. Stress and anxiety become important parameters to investigate.

All conditions that have already been considered in this chapter, together with diseases of cranial and peripheral nerves, must be excluded before making diagnosis of the facial pain dysfunction syndrome.

The basic component of the syndrome is functional disturbance of occlusion, muscle and joint.

Abnormalities of occlusion may act as initiators of sensory signals into a reflex system which will guide the mandible by means of muscle activity away from areas of painful premature dental contact. If the occlusal irregularity is slight and the patient's potential adaptive capacity towards pain is high, then a painless adjustment occurs readily. Severe malocclusion or continual stressful habits such as clenching or grinding the teeth, bruxism and/or posturing of the mandible, will result in persistent impulses to the muscles of mastication with possible tenderness, pain and dysfunction.

The muscles of mastication attempt to guide the mandible into an occlusal relationship of least interference and, in time, a position of occlusion is reached whereby the pain impulses are minimal. This is usually achieved at the expense of normal muscle function, and gives rise to abnormal or excessive normal movements and muscle fatigue.

The accumulation of metabolic products within fatigued muscle produces continuous recognizable pain.

Examination and Diagnostic Aids

The temporomandibular joint should be palpated and areas of tenderness noted. The degree of opening, together with abnormalities of function such as deviation either on opening or closing, should be recorded. The muscles of mastication should be palpated for areas of tenderness or hypertonicity which give rise to pain. The temporal, masseteric and digastric muscles may be palpated extra-orally whilst the pterygoid muscles may be palpated intra-orally. Individual muscle movement and function may be tested by observing muscle contraction during posturing movements.

Auscultation may be of value in detecting minor clicking and crepitous movement within the temporomandibular joint.

Local anaesthetic injections into particular muscles, external massage of muscles, and the application of ethyl chloride, ice or warmth may help to locate pain in the facial region more precisely.

A bite guard constructed of clear acrylic, with stainless steel clasps for retention, may prove not only of diagnostic but also of therapeutic help.

Prescribing drugs such as muscle relaxants, sedatives or tricyclic antidepressants is sometimes useful in patients exhibiting generalized muscle tension or psychosomatic anxiety symptoms.

The use of electromyography to register the electrical activity of the muscles of mastication may be of value. In the facial pain dysfunction syndrome patients appear to have excessive contractions and asymmetrical patterns of muscle activity.

Serological investigations help to exclude/include arthritic conditions of the temporomandibular joint, such as rheumatoid arthritis. This joint is usually affected late in the disease at a time when the classical stigmata of the condition are clinically obvious.

Treatment of the Facial Pain Dysfunction Syndrome

Essential treatment of dental, periodontal and occlusal abnormalities should be carried out. This may include restorations, work on dentures, and occlusal equilibration. The long-term use of a bite guard is of value for some patients. The majority of cases require reassurance, although a number may benefit from drug therapy such as sedatives and antidepressants. Intractable cases displaying marked emotional disturbance require psychiatric help, whilst recalcitrant cases may respond to injection of depot steroid into the joint.

FURTHER READING

Chalmers, I. M. & Blair, G. S. (1973) Rheumatoid arthritis of the temporomandibular joint. *Quarterly Journal of Medicine,* **42,** 369-386.
Toller, P. A. (1973) Osteoarthrosis of the mandibular condyle. *British Dental Journal,* **134,** 223-231.
Toller, P. A. (1974) Temporomandibular arthropathy. *Proceedings of the Royal Society of Medicine,* **67,** 153-159.

part 5

THE TEETH AND THE PERIODONTAL TISSUES IN SYSTEMIC DISEASE

chapter 19

Development, Structure and Function

The Structure of Teeth and Periodontal Tissues
The Development and Eruption of Teeth
The Function of Teeth and Periodontal Tissues

THE STRUCTURE OF TEETH AND PERIODONTAL TISSUES

The greater part of the mature tooth consists of dentine. The dentine is covered by enamel in the crown and by cementum in the root. Within the dentine is the pulp chamber containing the pulp tissue which consists of loose vascular connective tissue which is richly innervated.

The supporting tissues of the teeth consist of bone, cementum and periodontal membrane. The periodontal membrane consists mainly of collagenous fibres which constitute a suspensory ligament that attaches the tooth to the surrounding alveolar bone. The fibres are attached to the cementum and, for the most part, are inserted into the surrounding bone although some enter the gingival cuff region. The erupted tooth protrudes into the oral cavity through a cuff of mucous membrane (the gum or gingiva) which acts as a seal between the oral environment of the tooth crown and the underlying tissues of the tooth root and periodontium, that is, the bone, cementum and periodontal membrane.

On radiographic examination (Figure 19.1), the enamel (1) shows as an opaque white layer covering the crown, well demarcated from the cementum (2) and from the underlying dentine (3) which shows as a greyish layer in the crown and root surrounding the pulp chamber (4). The cortical layer of bone forming the tooth socket shows, as a radio-opaque line, the lamina dura (5). Between the root cementum and the lamina dura is the radiolucent periodontal membrane space.

THE DEVELOPMENT AND ERUPTION OF TEETH

The teeth start to develop at about six weeks in utero. A proliferation of the oral ectoderm, the primary epithelial band, divides into vestibular and dental laminae. A

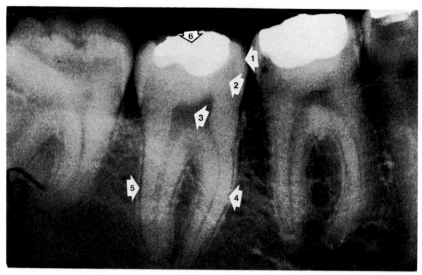

Figure 19.1. Periapical radiography of mandibular molar tooth, showing (1) enamel; (2) dentine; (3) pulp chamber; (4) cementum; (5) lamina dura; (6) filling.

downgrowth of the former results in formation of lips and cheeks and, from the latter, the teeth are subsequently formed from enamel organs, as shown diagrammatically in Figure 19.2a. Each enamel organ has an associated condensation of mesenchyme which is termed the 'dental papilla'. Between the enamel organ and dental papilla, the structures of the tooth are formed.

There are two major processes concerned in the development of the hard dental tissues, namely matrix formation and subsequent mineralization. In the inner layer of the enamel organ, the internal enamel epithelium (Figure 19.2b) maps out the form of the tooth crown and initiates the formation of dentine (dentinogenesis). Under its influence, the outer cells of the dental papilla form a layer of odontoblasts which deposit a layer of dentine. The cells of the inner enamel epithelium then shorten to become ameloblasts and thereafter enamel formation occurs (amelogenesis). The hard dental tissues thus separate the dental papilla from the enamel organ; the dental papilla becomes the dental pulp in the mature tooth. When the dentine in the root of the tooth begins to form, it is at first covered by the downgrowth of the external and internal enamel epithelia, the sheath of Hertwig. This maps out the root area of the tooth. After dentine formation has commenced, the epithelial sheath disintegrates but, long after eruption, the epithelial remains of Hertwig's sheath may be found lying between fibres of the periodontal membrane. They are known as the epithelial debris or rests of Malassez. Thus the surrounding connective tissue comes into contact with the dentine of the root and this induces those cells close to the dentine to differentiate into cementoblasts, which deposit cementum upon the root surface. When formation of the dentine and enamel of the tooth crown has been completed, the tooth moves towards the oral mucosa and erupts. The crown is covered by an epithelial layer derived from the enamel organ, the reduced enamel epithelium. On eruption, the latter fuses with the oral mucosa and, ultimately, the gingival crevice and epithelial attachment are formed. The root of the tooth is attached to the bone of the tooth socket by the periodontal membrane or ligament. It consists mainly of bundles of collagenous fibres passing from cementum to bone. The greater part of the mature tooth consists of dentine. The dentine is covered by enamel in the crown and by cementum in the root. Within the dentine is the pulp chamber containing the pulp tissue which consists of loose vascular connective tissue which is richly innervated.

Tables of approximate tooth formation and eruption dates for deciduous and permanent den.itions are shown in Table 19.1. This is a useful reference when considering possible deviations from the normal in systemic disease, where defects of tooth development, early or delayed eruption and prolonged retention of deciduous teeth may occur. It will be clear from Table 19.1 that a considerable variation and a large range of 'normal' exists among individuals.

Radiographic appearances of teeth and jaws vary with the age of the subject. Two stages of development are shown in Figures 19.3 (at six years of age) and 19.4 (at 14 years of age).

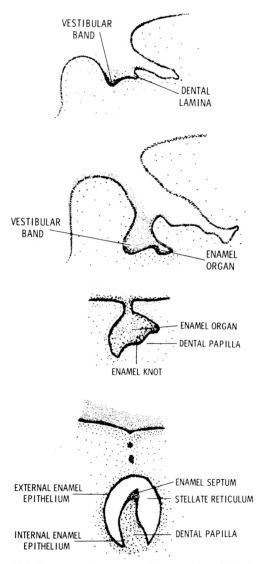

Figure 19.2. Diagrammatic representation of early tooth development.

Table 19.1. Chronology of tooth development.

	Tooth	Tooth germ fully formed	Dentine formation begins	Formation of crown complete	Appearance in mouth cavity	Root complete
Deciduous	Incisors			2–3 months	6–9 months	1–1½ years after appearance in mouth cavity
	Canines	3–4 months fetal life	4th–6th month fetal life	9 months	16–18 months	
	1st Molars			6 months	12–14 months	
	2nd Molars			12 months	20–30 months	
Permanent	Incisors	30th week fetal life	3–4 months (Upper lateral incisor 10–12 months)	4–5 years	Lower 6–8 years Upper 7–9 years	
	Canines	30th week fetal life	4–5 months	6–7 years	Lower 9–10 years Upper 11–12 years	2–3 years after appearance in mouth cavity
	Premolars	30th week fetal life	1½–2½ years	5–7 years	10–12 years	
	1st Molars	24th week fetal life	Before birth	2½–3 years	6–7 years	
	2nd Molars	6th month	2½–3 years	7–8 years	11–13 years	
	3rd Molars	6th year	7–10 years	12–16 years	17–21 years	

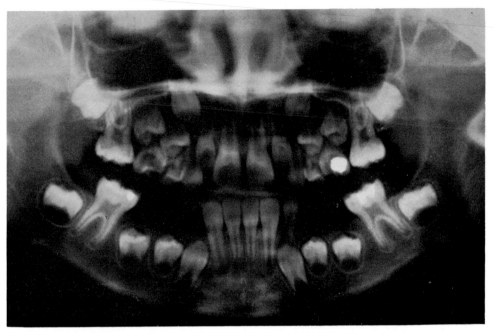

Figure 19.3. Normal dentition at the age of six years, shown radiographically.

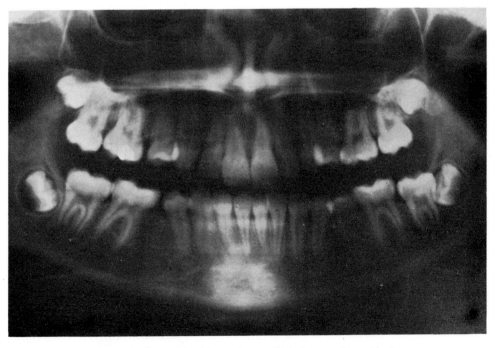

Figure 19.4. Normal dentition at the age of 14, shown radiographically.

THE FUNCTION OF TEETH AND PERIODONTAL TISSUES

There are many examples of teeth being malformed or hypoplastic due to systemic, nutritional or environmental influences during odontogenesis and some of these will be described in Chapter 20. However, the mature tooth, once formed, is subject only to minor changes in appearance, form or composition.

In contrast to the mature hard tooth tissues, the tissues of the periodontium, i.e., bone, periodontal membrane or ligament and cementum, once formed, are in a more dynamic metabolic state. Alveolar bone differs in no way from bone elsewhere in the body except that it is dependent for its existence on the presence of teeth. A continued process of resorption, apposition and remodelling occurs throughout life. Alveolar bone may become resorbed in relation to the pressure of tooth movement and permanent resorption occurs if the tooth is removed. Cementum, although a less active tissue than bone, also has the capacity for resorption, apposition and remodelling. The periodontal membrane, too, is capable of a high degree of functional adaptation and the collagen fibres show a moderately high degree of amino acid turnover.

Clearly, any of the known factors which regulate bone metabolism, such as dietary calcium, phosphate, vitamin D and hormones such as parathormone and calcitonin, may influence the alveolar bone in health and disease.

FURTHER READING

MacPhee, T. & Cowley, G. C. (1975) *Essentials of Periodontology and Periodontics,* 2nd ed. Oxford, London, Edinburgh, Melbourne: Blackwell Scientific Publications.

Scott, J. H. & Symons, N. B. B. (1961) *Introduction to Dental Anatomy.* Edinburgh and London: Churchill Livingstone.

Trapnell, D. H. & Bowerman, J. E. (1973) *Dental Manifestations of Systemic Disease. Radiology in Clinical Diagnoses Series.* London: Butterworth.

chapter 20

Dental Manifestations of Systemic Disease

Defective Development of Tooth Structure
Abnormalities Affecting Time of Eruption of Teeth
Changes in Mature Teeth after Eruption

DEFECTIVE DEVELOPMENT OF TOOTH STRUCTURE

During development, tooth structure may be influenced (a) during matrix formation, leading to hypoplasia and or hypomineralization, or (b) after formation but prior to eruption, leading to a degree of hypomineralization. These defects may be genetic in origin or may be the result of an environmental insult. Those due to an inherited fault may or may not be accompanied by other systemic manifestations but teeth are less frequently affected than bone. Generally speaking, gross skeletal defects are incompatible with life; as in osteogenesis imperfecta, for example, where there is a failure in bone matrix formation. Infants with the severe form of osteogenesis imperfecta congenita seldom survive and dentine formation is more severely affected than in osteogenesis imperfecta tarda, where the patient may have a normal life span.

Anodontia, partial anodontia, hypoplasia and/or hypocalcification, where enamel, dentine and cementum can be singly or collectively affected, are examples of defective tooth formation. These defects do not necessarily lead to increased dental decay or periodontal disease. For example, in partial anodontia, the enamel, dentine and cementum of the remaining teeth are normal and the tooth surfaces smooth. The teeth are usually widely spaced and many have a low incidence of caries. However, if the defect leads to a malocclusion, this will promote plaque accumulation, and will favour the common dental diseases such as caries and periodontitis.

Abnormalities of tooth structure or morphology (Figures 20.1 and 20.2) may be caused by genetic defects, chromosomal abnormalities, inborn errors of metabolism and a large and varied number of acquired systemic diseases, as detailed in Table 20.1. In this context, odontomes may be regarded as extreme examples of abnormality which often have a genetic basis.

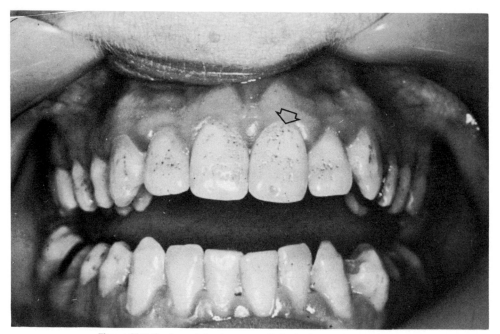

Figure 20.1. Surface pitting in a case of inherited enamel hypoplasia.

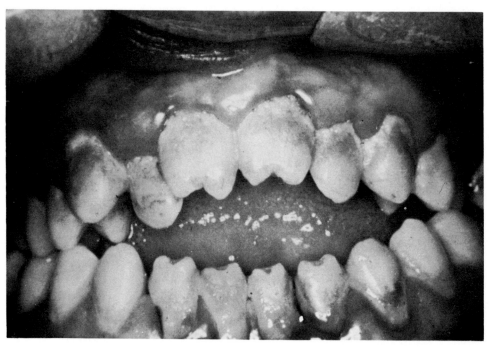

Figure 20.2. The characteristic notching of the incisal teeth in a case of prenatal syphilis.

Table 20.1.

Enamel hypoplasia

Mongolism	Tetracycline therapy
Phenylketonuria	Hypervitaminosis D
Exanthematous fevers	Hypothyroidism
Sickle cell anaemia	Hypoparathyroidism
Neonatal haemolytic anaemia	Diabetes mellitus
Rickets	Nephrotic syndrome
Epidermolysis bullosa	Ehlers — Danlos syndrome
Fluorosis	

Dentinal hypoplasia
　Dentinogenesis Imperfecta
　Hypoparathyroidism
　Ehlers — Danlos syndrome

Cemental hypoplasia
　Hypophosphatasia
　Cleidocranial dysostosis

Cemental hyperplasia
　Age
　Paget's disease of bone
　Hyperpituitarism

Premature eruption
　Extraction of deciduous precursor
　Hyperpituitarism
　Adrenogenital syndrome

Delayed eruption
　Local factors, e.g. malocclusion, cysts, odontomes
　Rickets
　Irradiation
　Hypopituitarism
　Hypoparathyroidism
　Hypothyroidism
　Cleidocranial dysostosis

ABNORMALITIES AFFECTING TIME OF ERUPTION OF TEETH

The eruption time of teeth is frequently affected by local factors although, rarely, certain systemic disorders may also influence eruption.

Premature eruption of deciduous or permanent teeth may occur in such endocrine disturbances as adrenogenital syndrome, hyperthyroidism or hyperpituitarism. Delayed eruption of deciduous or permanent teeth may occur in cretinism or hypo-thyroidism and hypopituitarism, rickets and cleidocranial dysostosis (Figure 20.3). In the latter, it is usually the permanent teeth which are affected.

CHANGES IN MATURE TEETH AFTER ERUPTION

The loss of tooth surface due to attrition and abrasion is well known. Certain biochemical changes such as decalcification and remineralization occur on the enamel surface and, although these are mainly related to local dietary and salivary constituents, occasionally they may be the result of systemic disease elsewhere; for example, acid regurgitation in chronic gastritis can cause tooth erosion.

Little is known about changes which might occur via the pulp tissue but it would appear that these are extremely rare.

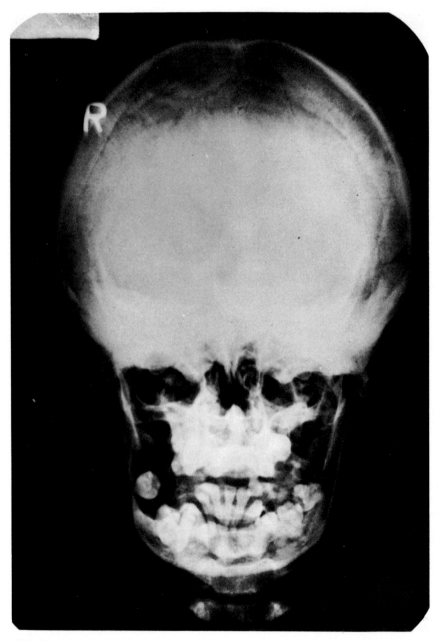

Figure 20.3. Retention of deciduous teeth and delayed eruption of permanent teeth in a patient aged 14 years with cleidocranial dysostosis. Other typical changes are present in the skull.

Abrasion, Attrition and Erosion

Loss of tooth surface may occur by three separate processes: abrasion, attrition and erosion.

Abrasion is related to an external mechanical factor, such as the incorrect use of a toothbrush, particularly in combination with an abrasive dentifrice (Figure 20.4).

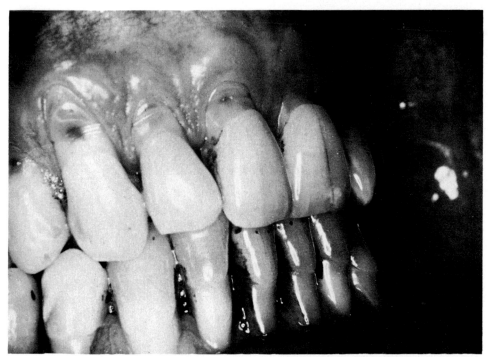

Figure 20.4. An example of toothbrush abrasion showing exposed dentine at the cervical margins of the teeth.

Attrition is the wearing away of the tooth surface through intertooth contact (Figure 20.5). It may be caused by bruxism which, in turn, may be related to some underlying stress, mood disorder or psychiatric disturbance. Further causes of excessive attrition are the inclusion of excessive roughage in the diet and abnormalities of tooth structure. Attrition is also a marker of age.

Erosion can be defined as the loss of tooth substance by a chemical process and, unlike dental caries, does not include bacterial action (Figure 20.6). It may be observed in patients who have certain food fads, such as the habitual sucking of lemons or the drinking of acidic beverages. It may also be observed as a complication of some systemic diseases where excessive vomiting or acid regurgitation is a recurrent feature. The pattern of tooth loss will differ according to the source; for example, the lingual and palatal surfaces with acid regurgitation, and the labial surfaces with acid fumes. The latter may be seen in workers who handle concentrated acids.

Management. Identification of the cause and its removal, where possible, is indicated. Systemic factors causing attrition can be complex but have to be considered along with the taking of local measures, such as balancing occlusion. Night splints may be necessary in the treatment of bruxism. Fissure sealants, such as Nuva Seal, have a valuable role in the treatment of eroded surfaces regardless of their cause.

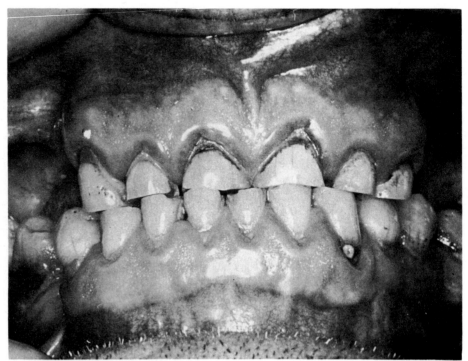

Figure 20.5. Marked loss of tooth substance (attrition) by patient who is an habitual bruxist.

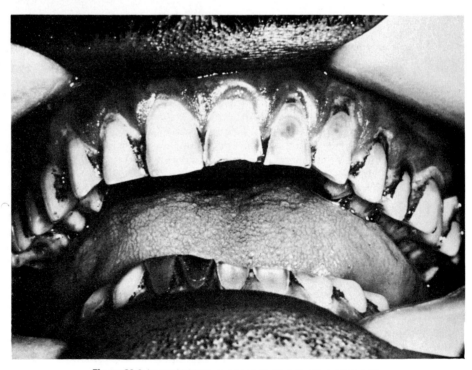

Figure 20.6. Loss of labial enamel and dentine due to erosion only.

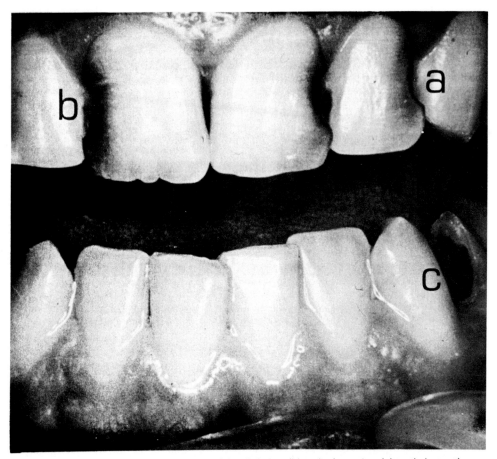

Figure 20.7. Dental caries at various stages: (a) early lesion; (b) cavity formation; (c) tooth destruction.

Dental Caries and Periodontal Disease

The main dental diseases are caries and periodontitis (Figures 20.7 and 20.8). Both are pandemic and, in both, the dominant aetiological factors are local and intra-oral. Additionally, in otherwise normal patients there is wide variation in the severity of both caries and periodontal disease. For example, a young child may have grossly carious teeth and established gingivitis, while an elderly adult may be fully dentate, caries free, and with a healthy periodontum, despite the fact that the adult's teeth have been exposed to important aetiological factors for many more years. The identification of systemic conditions which affect the natural course of dental caries and periodontal disease, if they exist at all, is difficult. This is exemplified in mongolism (Down's syndrome) where complicating factors of mental retardation, often resulting in poor oral hygiene and unfavourable diet, institutionalization of the patient and delayed eruption time of the teeth all influence the exposure of the dental tissues to the risk of dental disease. Therefore, in order to establish whether or not the systemic condition (Down's syndrome) is influencing the natural course of dental disease, it is necessary to compare patients with mongolism, not only with normal subjects, but also with other mental defectives, and to compare institutionalized patients with subjects (siblings, for example) who live in the home environment.

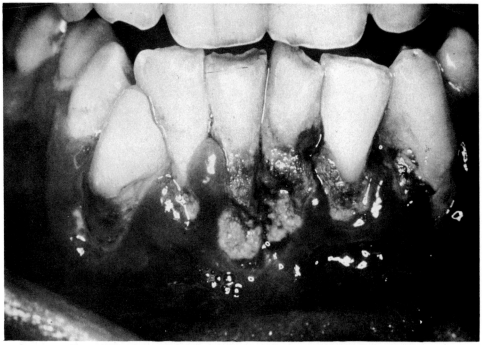

Figure 20.8. Advanced periodontal disease with gross calculus and pocketing.

Handicaps, both physical and mental, customarily result in poor oral hygiene and increased severity of dental disease entirely due to the local factors. A temporary lapse in oral hygiene with resultant increased plaque accumulation may arise, for instance, in a patient with a broken arm, or facial palsy leading to unilateral chewing and eating with neglect of oral hygiene on the affected side. In conditions of greater duration and severity, such as congenital myotonic dystrophy, where the muscle tone is affected, malocclusion may result and these patients may also have mental retardation, all mitigating against a satisfactory level of oral hygiene. Management of these patients often requires a team effort.

It is not clear whether teeth with defective enamel and or dentine are, per se, more susceptible to caries than are clinically normal teeth; important factors seem to be the site of the defect, that is, whether it is in a region of the tooth where plaque accumulates readily; the degree of mineralization; and the integrity of the amelodental junction which, when weakened, can give rise to fractured enamel. Once teeth have erupted, systemic conditions may influence the carious process through the local factors, saliva, gingival fluid and the intra-oral influence of diet.

The local aetiological factor common to both caries and periodontal disease is the metabolic activity of the bacteria resident in the dental plaque. However, the target tissues differ in their response to the noxious stimulant. In caries, the enamel surface is the target tissue and is, in itself, inert although some recalcification may occur from saliva. In periodontal disease the tissues are vital and the full range of systemic response to tissue damage may be mobilized.

It has long been recognized that saliva is a major, post-eruptive, intrinsic determinant in the carious process. A direct relationship can be shown between salivary flow rate and caries incidence when large numbers of patients are investigated. There is some evidence that a high buffering capacity, alkaline pH and optimum concentrations

Table 20.2. *Mechanisms and conditions which may cause reduced salivation.*

Gland	Sjögren's syndrome
	Post-irradiation
Neural	VII and IX cranial nerve lesions
	Superior cervical ganglion lesion
	Reduced taste perception
Hormonal	Diabetes mellitus
Emotional	Depression
Drugs	e.g., CNS depressants;
	hypotensive agents;
	antihistamines

of calcium and phosphorus predispose to a low level of decay and this is entirely compatible with the acidogenic theory of caries. Additionally, the activity of anti-bacterial factors in saliva would be expected to affect the microbial composition of plaque.

Therefore, conditions in which the secretion of saliva is affected (see Table 20.2) would be expected to have an affect on caries and periodontal disease. The classic example is xerostomia due to Sjögren's syndrome, where the onset of salivary gland disease is accompanied by a rapid increase in caries activity (Figure 20.9) and periodontal destruction.

Altered salivary secretions are found both in mongolism and cystic fibrosis. An increase in calcium and buffering capacity and, probably, salivary IgA in cystic fibrosis has been seen associated with increased calculus formation and gingivitis.

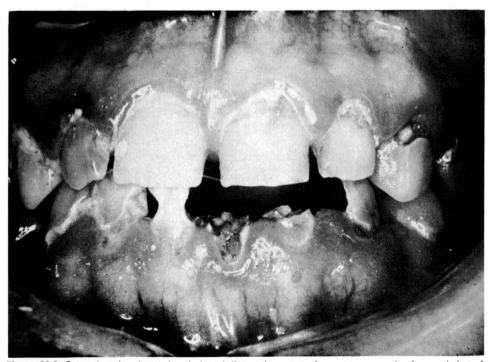

Figure 20.9. Gross dental caries and periodontal disease in a case of severe xerostomia. Accumulation of plaque and the rapid onset of smooth surface caries occur typically in patients with decreased salivary function.

Recent studies in mongolism using appropriate controls, as discussed above, have demonstrated a lower than normal level of caries. This, too, may be attributable to increased salivary calcium and buffering capacity. The caries level in patients with cystic fibrosis does not seem to have been thoroughly investigated.

The antibacterial factors in saliva would be expected to regulate the commensal flora. No systemic conditions appear to have been reported in which salivary lysozyme, lactoferrin or the peroxidase thiocyanate systems are altered. However, the caries and periodontal status of a few patients with IgA deficiency have been studied but no definite trend has been established.

Systemic conditions where the patient's diet, in particular carbohydrate consumption, is markedly altered, will affect caries incidence. As a general principle, if carbohydrates, which are readily fermentable by the bacteria of dental plaque, are consumed frequently and in large quantities, there is a high rate of dental caries. In two rare but interesting conditions, in which there is an inborn error of metabolism, there is a markedly low level of dental caries. These conditions are hereditary fructose intolerance and congenital sucrose deficiency where the affected subjects cannot tolerate sucrose and where the carbohydrate source in the diet is usually starch.

Considering periodontal disease per se, most otherwise normal patients present with non-specific gingivitis which, if untreated, may progress to non-specific periodontitis. A very small number of patients present with periodontosis (rapid periodontal destruction not commensurate with the degree of local irritation). The other common periodontal condition is acute ulcerative gingivitis, where the histopathological feature is necrosis. Considerable evidence exists to suggest that this specific condition, which is accompanied by an increase in the proportion of fusiform bacilli and spirochaetes, also has an important systemic factor of altered host—parasite balance. Stress and smoking have both been shown to increase the susceptibility to acute ulcerative gingivitis (Figure 20.10). Whether this is due to reduced oxygenation of the tip of the inderdental papilla or an altered immune response, or both, requires further investigation.

Increased susceptibility to periodontal disease has been suggested in a variety of conditions, such as pregnancy, leukaemia, diabetes mellitus and in patients receiving drugs, e.g. phenytoin and contraceptive pill.

Of these, pregnancy gingivitis (Figure 20.11) is by far the most common condition and to some extent gingivitis presents in the majority of pregnant women examined.

It is suggested that in pregnancy some other factor is present which, together with bacterial plaque, may be responsible for accentuating inflammatory changes in the gingiva. It may be that increase in the permeability of the ground substance which occurs as a result of changes in the levels of circulating sex hormones during pregnancy may lead to exacerbation of pre-existing inflammation in the presence of dental plaque. Accordingly, pregnant females should be urged to increase their level of oral hygiene.

The gingiva reverts to a normal prepregnant condition (Figure 20.12) shortly after parturition and surgical intervention is rarely necessary.

Leukaemia and diabetes mellitus may be associated with an increased susceptibility to gingivitis and periodontal disease and these subjects have been dealt with in detail in Chapters 7 and 8 respectively.

Dental treatment for patients with increased dental disease attributable to systemic conditions should be aimed primarily at prevention, through improved oral hygiene, control of dietary sugar, the use of fluorides and other preventive measures, such as fissure sealants. However, in cases where oral hygiene cannot be brought to an adequate level and focal sepsis might endanger life, or continued rapid bone loss make the subsequent provision of dentures difficult, early extraction should be considered.

It is not surprising that early in some systemic diseases the bone of the tooth socket, i.e. the lamina dura as shown on a radiograph may show evidence of change such as

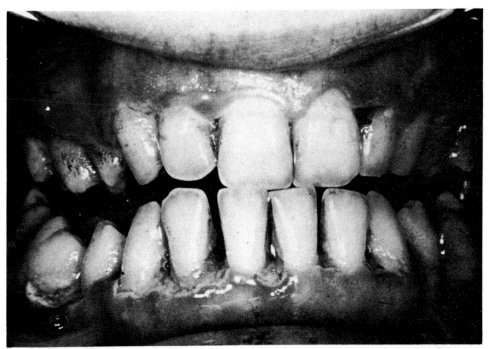

Figure 20.10. Typical ulceration of the gingival papillae in a patient with acute ulcerative gingivitis (Vincent's type).

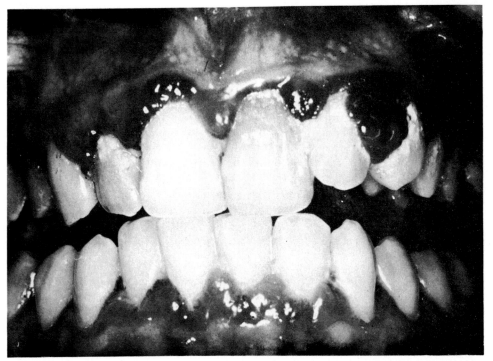

Figure 20.11. Inflammatory swelling and bleeding of the gingiva in a typical case of pregnancy gingivitis.

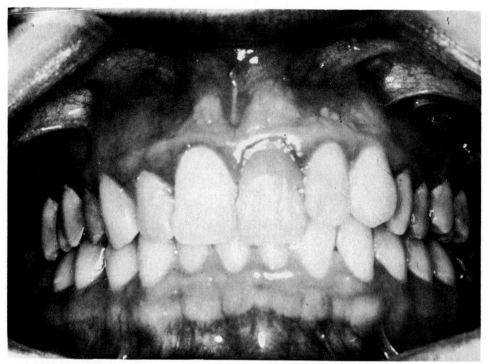

Figure 20.12. Appearance of patient in Figure 20.11 three months postpartum showing complete remission of gingivitis.

increased radiolucency in hyperparathyroidism or increased density in osteopetrosis. In the early phase of Paget's disease there can be both increased apposition and increased resorption of alveolar bone and cementum and, in the later stages, excessive deposition of both bone and cementum may occur.

In conclusion, systemic conditions which effect dental disease are uncommon but, as the level of prevention in the general population improves, these conditions may become more apparent. Additionally, as medical science prolongs the life of patients who suffer from the rare conditions discussed above, more of these patients will be seeking dental treatment. Dental management of such cases requires early and accurate diagnosis. Detailed study of the mechanisms by which systemic conditions effect dental disease may be a useful research tool to increase our understanding of caries and periodontal disease.

FURTHER READING

Mergenhagen, S. E. & Scherp, H. W. (Eds.) (1973) *Comparative Immunology of the Oral Cavity,* D.H.E.W. Publication No. (NIH) 73/438. Bethesda, Maryland: U.S. Department of Health, Education and Welfare, Public Health Service.

Poole, A. E. (Ed.) (1975) Symposium on Genetics, *The Dental Clinics of North America,* **19**, (1).

Stanbury, J. B., Wyngaarden, J. B. & Fredrickson, D. S. (Eds.) (1972) *The Metabolic Basis of Inherited Disease,* 3rd ed. New York: McGraw-Hill.

part 6

DISEASE OF THE
NERVOUS SYSTEM

Neurological Disease

INTRODUCTION

Many diseases of the nervous system and muscles produce oral symptoms and signs, which are comparatively few in number in contrast to the large variety of the diseases which may be at fault. In the present chapter, diseases have been classified under the symptoms or signs they produce.

It is not the object of this chapter to provide coverage of the whole field of neurology, but it will give examples of the major groups of disorders which have oral manifestations. Early in the course of some of the diseases to be described patients may have bizarre complaints which cannot easily be related to each other, and the disease may be identified wrongly as a 'psychiatric' disturbance.

When considering the symptom of pain it is important to evaluate the individual personality along with the patient's social and ethnic background. A knowledge of a patient's personality prior to his developing a painful disorder enables the clinician to predict how he will behave when in pain and his potential response to treatment, as well as to estimate the psychological changes which occur consequential to pain.

CLINICAL EXAMINATION OF THE NERVOUS SYSTEM IN THE MOUTH AND ADJACENT TISSUES

A complete description of the examination of all the cranial nerves is outside the scope of this text and standard medical texts should be consulted. The following cranial nerves will be discussed: V, VII, IX, X and XII.

Trigeminal Nerve

Lesions of the ophthalmic division result in loss of sensation in the skin of forehead, and part of the nose and upper eyelid as well as the conjunctiva.

Sensation is tested by asking the patient to close his eyes and report each time that he feels the appropriate region being touched. Total anaesthesia is not always the rule and it may be found that when a sharp point is used the patient can appreciate only that he is being touched but be unable to discriminate between sharp and blunt probes.

The maxillary division supplies the skin of cheeks, upper lip, side of nose and nasal mucosa, upper teeth and gingivae, palatal mucosa and upper labial mucosa. Disorders affecting this branch of the trigeminal nerve result in a loss of sensation in these areas and may also produce a loss of the palatal reflex.

The mandibular division, in addition to supplying the skin of the lower face, lower teeth and gingivae, tongue and floor of mouth, also has a motor supply to the muscles of mastication. Lesions of the mandibular division lead to a loss of sensation in the appropriate areas of skin and mucosa. Touch, but not taste, to the lingual mucosa is affected.

The muscles of mastication are tested by asking the patient to open and then to clench the jaw; no deviation should occur and both masseters can be palpated. In addition, the jaw should be moved laterally as well as protruded.

Facial Nerve

The facial nerve supplies most of the muscles of the face (excluding the muscles of mastication) as well as the submandibular and sublingual salivary glands. In addition, it is also responsible for taste from the anterior two-thirds of tongue by way of the chorda tympani.

The facial nerve is tested by asking the patient sequentially to raise his eyebrows, to screw the eyes tightly shut, to whistle, to smile and show his teeth. The patient inflates his mouth by blowing the cheeks out and attempts to keep the lips closed. Each cheek is tapped and if there is weakness to one side then air will escape much more readily when that side is tapped.

A distinction can often be made between upper and lower motor neurone involvement. In supranuclear lesions it is mainly the lower half of the face which is affected as there is a bilateral innervation to the forehead and a unilateral lesion cuts off impulses only from some of the supply.

In contrast, a lesion below the nucleus results in both the upper and lower halves of the face being equally affected.

Taste will be diminished in lesions of the seventh cranial nerve and this should be tested by applying the four gustatory stimuli to the dorsum of the tongue. The following are appropriate:

Sour   — citric acid solution
Salt   — salt solution
Sweet — sucrose solution
Bitter — quinine or gentian solution

It is thought that some taste fibres may also run with the trigeminal nerve, although this is variable.

The orifices of the submandibular and sublingual salivary glands are on the floor of the mouth, and the flow of saliva from each orifice should be noted and compared following the application of a strong gustatory stimulus, for example 10 per cent aqueous citric acid. (This is, of course, only valid in the presence of an intact sense of taste on some part of the tongue.)

Glossopharyngeal Nerve

The ninth cranial nerve supplies sensation and taste to the posterior one-third of tongue as well as sensation to the pharyngeal mucosa. In addition, the glosso-pharyngeal nerve has motor branches to the parotid salivary gland and the middle pharyngeal constrictor.

This nerve is tested by taste on the posterior third of tongue and by touching the pharyngeal mucosa and observing the reflex action.

The parotid orifice is on the buccal mucosa and, again, the flow of saliva from right and left sides should be compared after applying a gustatory stimulus to the tongue.

Vagus Nerve

The tenth cranial nerve has motor and sensory connections to a number of thoracic and abdominal viscera: the only aspect under consideration in the present text, however, is its innervation to the muscles of the soft palate.

Separate lesions of the ninth, tenth or eleventh nerve are uncommon and one usually finds a degree of involvement of all three.

The oral component of the vagus nerve is tested by asking about problems during swallowing (due to defective elevation of the soft palate), with regurgitation into the nose.

The soft palate is observed and the patient asked to say 'Ah'. Both sides of the soft palate should arch up symmetrically and the uvula should remain central. Should there be a lesion affecting the vagus nerve, the uvula will deviate to the opposite side of the lesion and the same side of the soft palate will not be elevated.

Hypoglossal Nerve

The twelfth nerve supplies the muscles of the tongue and depressors of the hyoid bone. In order to test the hypoglossal nerve the patient is asked to protrude the tongue. If the tongue deviates, it is being pushed towards the paralysed side. On examination, the affected side may show evidence of muscle wasting and the patient is unable to move the tongue from side to side.

NEUROLOGICAL DISORDERS AS A CAUSE OF ORAL PAIN

Patients often find difficulty in precise localization of oral pain and may indicate a vague area of the face as the site of their complaint. Facial pain may originate in many structures and these are listed in convenient groups below.

1. Dental and periodontal structures.
2. The jaw bones.
3. The temporomandibular joint and associated muscles.
4. The facial soft tissues, including the oral mucous membrane.

5. The paranasal sinuses, nose, ears and throat.
6. The eyes.
7. The heart and blood vessels.
8. The nervous system, including the mind.

The section which follows deals primarily with pain originating from diseases of the nervous system, but some other disorders, such as migraine, which have a vascular basis are included for convenience.

Trigeminal Neuralgia (Tic Douloureux)

Trigeminal neuralgia occurs as episodic, recurrent, unilateral facial pain which affects the right side more often than the left, and usually persons of more than 50 years of age. Women are affected more frequently than men. The pain may affect any of the areas supplied by the branches of the fifth cranial nerve and recurrent episodes sometimes involve a different branch or side of the face. The pain comes spontaneously, or may be triggered by a stimulus, such as touch or movement. Thus, patients may point to the site of the pain, conspicuously holding the pointing finger 1 cm away from the skin, terrified lest touch may trigger a new episode of pain; or one half of the tongue may be coated because it is not moved or used in mastication, or one half of the face may not be shaven. The pain, which is excruciating, comes in high intensity jabs, each lasting 20 to 30 seconds and separated by a brief respite.

The pain rarely spreads beneath the ramus of the mandible or behind the ear. There is no disturbance in motor function or of sensation. During an attack, the affected half of the face takes on a cramped expression and the cheek may become red. The spasms of pain come with variable frequency for periods of a few months, though seldom during sleep, and remissions of several months are commonplace. The diagnosis of trigeminal neuralgia should not be made in young patients or in patients with motor or sensory dysfunction without a most careful neurological assessment.

The cause of trigeminal neuralgia is not known but there is strong presumptive evidence to suggest that the pain originates in disturbed function in the peripheral neurones of the trigeminal system. Degenerative changes have been demonstrated in certain nerve fibres from the face and mouth which provide an inhibitory influence on relays through the spinal nucleus of the trigeminal nerve. However, while the disorder is likely to be due to loss of inhibition of the flow of nociceptive afferent discharges through the spinal nucleus of the fifth nerve, this effect may be produced by mechanisms in the peripheral or central portions of the system, and the degenerative changes referred to above may represent only one of several possible mechanisms.

Trigeminal neuralgia responds in many patients to the administration of carbamazepine (Tegretol) in doses of 100 to 200 mg once or twice daily. This dose may require to be increased slowly to levels of 400 to 600 mg, and above, per day to achieve a suitable response. The drug should not be used with monoaminoxidase inhibitors or within two weeks of the use of these drugs. It is wise, also, to monitor the peripheral blood during prolonged use of the drug.

Glossopharyngeal Neuralgia

Glossopharyngeal neuralgia is less common than trigeminal neuralgia. It occurs in middle-aged patients as a paroxysmal pain localized in the tonsil, back of the tongue or ear. The pain is variously described as burning or stabbing in character and may be triggered by swallowing, moving the tongue, talking or touch. During attacks, patients sometimes feel faint or lose consciousness. There is no loss of sensation or of motor power. The pain can vary in frequency of occurrence from several times per day to once in several weeks and there may be prolonged remissions.

Post-herpetic Neuralgia

Pain is a characteristic feature of herpes zoster and usually precedes the appearance of the skin rash. The pain subsides in a few weeks in young patients but may persist for months or indefinitely in older patients, particularly in those of 70 years and over. The pain is steady and sustained and is described as burning or boring. Alteration in sensation and muscular weakness may be associated with post-herpetic neuralgia.

The diagnosis of post-herpetic neuralgia is indicated by a history of herpes zoster.

Migraine

Migraine is a periodic headache which occasionally involves the face and neck. More often the pain is temporal or supra-orbital in site but it may affect the malar region or the upper or lower teeth. Attacks tend to be preceded by a feeling of buoyancy and exhilaration. This is followed by prodromal symptoms which may be visual, sensory, or other, such as speech disturbance. The headache is at first unilateral and throbbing in character but becomes generalized and aching. It is associated with irritability, photophobia, nausea and vomiting and the patient looks and feels ill. The attack is usually completed in the course of one day (sun-up to sundown) and is followed, as it was preceded, by a feeling of well-being. There is often a family history, with mother and daughter being victims of the same disorder. The prodromal symptoms are probably due to a phase of vasoconstriction preceding vasodilation which causes the headache and associated phenomena. Treatment is by ergot and similar drugs.

Periodic Migrainous Neuralgia

Periodic migrainous neuralgia, also called cluster headache, occurs as bouts of high-intensity boring pain, sited unilaterally around the eye or in the temple, face, upper or lower teeth or neck. The attacks last for about one hour and often occur at night, wakening the patient with alarm-clock regularity at the same time on each of several nights in succession. Affected patients are usually in middle or old age and during an attack they experience unilateral watering and congestion of the eye and nose. There is apparent perspiration and the skin overlying the cheek on the affected side becomes red. Severely affected patients may experience the pain at intervals of a few hours night and day for months.

Periodic migrainous neuralgia may be differentiated from trigeminal neuralgia by its failure to follow the distribution of the fifth cranial nerve and its branches and by the absence of a trigger mechanism. The bouts of pain are also longer. Nausea and vomiting do not occur as in migraine and there are no prodromal symptoms. The attacks usually last about one hour, in contrast to the sun-up—sundown duration of migraine. Nevertheless, it is thought that this form of neuralgia, like migraine, is due to vascular phenomena.

Conditions which Mimic Trigeminal Neuralgia

Certain diseases of the nervous system produce neuralgic symptoms which may mimic trigeminal neuralgia as described above. It is most important that the true nature of these be recognized, since failure to do so may result in incorrect treatment or lack of treatment of some condition requiring surgical intervention.

In young patients, and particularly where the pain persists between spasms, the possibility of multiple sclerosis should be considered.

Tumours in the region of the trigeminal ganglion, in the cranium (usually metastatic deposits from carcinomas elsewhere in the body), in the middle fossa and in the cerebellopontine angle may cause painful jabs in the face. Usually, in these cases, the pain persists for several minutes and there may be anaesthesia of part of the face. Often other facial nerves are affected, producing a variety of other signs and symptoms.

Atypical Facial Pain

A number of patients complain of neuralgic pain which persists for hours or days and which is not triggered. Often these patients are younger than is usual for neuralgia and the pain is diffuse, affecting areas outside those supplied by the fifth cranial nerve. These cases present a difficult diagnostic problem but it is important to identify or exclude any dental cause for the pain. This requires most careful dental assessment. If there is no dental cause, other organic disease should be excluded by appropriate investigation, which may include neurological and psychiatric assessment.

It should be noted that trigeminal neuralgia may present with atypical features and some time may elapse before the usual characteristics of this disorder appear.

Chronic Post-Traumatic Headache

Patients who have suffered head injury often complain of persistent headache for some time afterwards. This headache may be localized to the site of the injury, or be described as a sensation of pressure or band-like constriction. Some patients experience a throbbing, aching pain which occurs in bouts and often on one side only. Such pain may result from local tissue damage or from other ill effects following trauma. However, often there is no such pathological change. Apprehension, fear, resentment and other emotional reactions are commonplace, and understandable, after head injury, particularly where a highly intellectual patient fears deterioration in mental capacity after such an injury: this apprehension may cause tension and exacerbate or prolong the symptoms caused by the trauma. Such patients require careful supervision and the care of a neurologist.

NEUROLOGICAL DISORDERS AS A CAUSE OF ANAESTHESIA

Facial anaesthesia is an important sign which, if not due to disease within the jaw bones or to dental procedures such as the extraction of a tooth or needle trauma, necessitates further examination and investigation. The causes of facial anaesthesia are listed below:

1. Dental treatment, e.g. removal of impacted mandibular third molar teeth, or of other teeth, or needle trauma.
2. Neoplasms, cysts or other disease within the jaws or facial bones.
3. Neoplasms in the nasopharynx.
4. Viral infections such as herpes zoster which may present with numbness.
5. Collagen diseases, such as disseminated lupus erythematosus, periarteritis nodosa and dermatomyositis, which may affect nerves.
6. Demyelinating diseases of the nervous system, such as disseminated sclerosis.
7. Tumours of the brain and intracranial tumours.
8. Psychiatric disorders.

A careful history is required to exclude dental treatment or disease as a cause of the anaesthesia. Examination will indicate which division of the trigeminal nerve is affected but in patients with psychiatric disease the anaesthesia may bear no relationship to the distribution of the branches of this nerve. Clinical and radiographic examination will assist in the excluding of other causes within the mouth or mandible. Diagnosis of the neurological disorders referred to above requires proper assessment of the nervous system. The reader is referred to the texts given under Further Reading at the end of this chapter for a full account of this.

NEUROLOGICAL DISORDERS AS A CAUSE OF FACIAL PARALYSIS

Inability to perform voluntary movements may result from many disorders, as follows:

1. Disease of the cerebral cortex results in inability to formulate and utilize movements previously easily undertaken. There is no actual paralysis but the patient may make bizarre mistakes in performing simple movements.
2. Disease lower in the brain or in the spinal cord causes disturbance of the upper motor neurone and paralysis, spasticity and a peculiar rhythmic series of muscular contractions, referred to as clonus, when a muscle is passively stretched.
3. Damage of the nerve cells in the anterior horns of the spinal cord, or of the peripheral nerve, disrupts the lower motor neurone and causes wasting and weakness of the muscles supplied by that nerve. Spontaneous contractions may occur in such muscles (fibrillation or fasciculation) and there is loss of muscle tone.
4. Disturbance of function at the neuromuscular junction, such as occurs in myasthenia gravis, causes weakness and excessive fatiguability.
5. Primary disease of muscle causes wasting and weakness of muscles.
6. Disorders of the extrapyramidal pathways and of the cerebellum cause delay and reduction in the amplitude of movements, disturbances of tone and involuntary movements.

Examples of the oral manifestations of some of the above are given in the sections that follow.

Upper Motor Neurone Paralysis

Obstruction of a cerebral artery will result in infarction of the part of the brain supplied by that artery. A variety of signs and symptoms results, depending on the site and cause of the infarct. Weakness of the face, tongue, dysphagia, facial pain and paraesthesia can occur, but these oral manifestations are usually overshadowed by other signs of the stroke, such as extensive paralysis. The patient is unlikely to seek dental advice and the dentist meeting such complaints is hardly likely to imagine they are due to dental disease.

Upper and Lower Motor Neurone Paralysis

This paralysis occurs in amyotrophic lateral sclerosis and is caused by degenerative changes in the medulla and spinal cord. Such changes produce progressive wasting of muscles. On rare occasions, patients with this disorder present to the dentist complaining of inability to eat properly, but this is usually associated with inability to speak. The tongue may show small involuntary movements called fasciculations and food may be ejected from the mouth, or into the nose, during swallowing.

Lower Motor Neurone Paralysis

Bilateral lower motor neurone facial palsy may occur in acute post-infective polyneuritis (the Guillain—Barré syndrome) about 10 to 14 days after an acute infection such as influenza. Such patients have difficulty in chewing and may complain of a feeling of heaviness in the jaw. The dentist may be misled by such bizarre complaints and may fail to detect the paralysis, or he may imagine that the patient's failure to move the jaw is a manifestation of tetanus. Immediate referral to a physician is required so that suitable treatment may result in a return to normal function.

Unilateral lower motor neurone facial paralysis occurs as Bell's palsy. This is a common disease and may affect all ages and both sexes. Patients usually complain of pain behind the ear, and of feeling unwell before the onset of the palsy, which is abrupt and reaches its maximum within one day. Recovery is possible in a few weeks but, particularly in older patients, the paralysis may be permanent.

The diagnosis may be apparent from the facial asymmetry and flattening of the facial grooves visible on inspection of the face. However, when the paralysis has been present for some time the muscles undergo contracture so that the facial grooves may be deeper on the paralysed than on the normal side. Diagnosis can be made when the patient is requested to move the face and the paralysis will be demonstrated when the patient is commanded to whistle, purse the lips, firmly close the eyes and wrinkle the forehead. When the patient attempts to close the eye, the eyeball will move upwards so that the pupil is hidden beneath the upper eyelid although the eye is not closed. This phenomenon (Bell's phenomenon) occurs in lower motor neurone lesions of the seventh nerve, and is not a feature of disturbance of the upper motor neurone.

Treatment by corticosteroids within 24 hours of the onset of the paralysis may improve the chances for recovery. Otherwise the exposed eye must be protected and, in the long term, plastic, prosthetic or neurosurgical procedures may be considered to correct the facial deformity.

Unilateral lower motor neurone facial paralysis may also result from trauma to the facial nerve or by malignant tumours in the parotid gland. Such causes may result in paralysis of some of the muscles on the affected side, and other muscles may escape.

Disorders of Neuromuscular Transmission

Disorders of neuromuscular transmission, such as myasthenia gravis, are characterized by abnormal fatiguability of striated muscle and patients usually present with ptosis (drooping of the eyelids) which causes an appearance of sleepiness. Weakness of the facial muscles produces an apathetic, expressionless appearance and the patient may find difficulty in speaking and swallowing. Tiring of the muscles occurs on mastication and the patient is left with the mouth hanging open and the teeth widely apart.

Disorders of Muscle

Myasthenia, or muscle weakness, occurs as a symptom in polymyositis, systemic lupus erythematosus, dermatomyositis and in some forms of carcinomatous myopathy. Patients with the latter have presented with difficulty in talking, chewing and closing the mouth. Some have found it necessary to assist chewing with the hand. Symptoms such as these are cause for a comprehensive health check and cannot be ascribed to dental disease.

NEUROLOGICAL DISORDERS AS A CAUSE OF INCREASED MUSCLE TONE OR ABNORMAL MUSCLE MOVEMENTS

Tetanus

The early symptoms of tetanus, trismus, dysphagia and neck stiffness draw attention to the mouth and, in error, may be ascribed to dental disease. The patient may fail to report a recent wound, or may have forgotten the incident. The diagnosis is all the more difficult in those cases where the disease has followed a facial or an intra-oral wound, since under these circumstances the symptoms of tetanus are likely to be attributed to a direct effect of the wound. Nevertheless, tetanus should be considered in the differential diagnosis of trismus, particularly when intra-oral causes are lacking or insignificant.

Muscle Disorders

Some muscular dystrophies are associated with alteration in muscle tone. An example is *myotonic muscular dystrophy* which is characterized by increased muscle tone, muscular atrophy which particularly affects the face and neck, cataracts, premature frontal hair loss and endocrine dysfunction, including testicular atrophy. The disease is inherited. With this disease, muscles fail to relax after forceful contraction. The patient has a dull expressionless appearance with ptosis and muscular atrophy; and frontal hair loss accentuates the 'hatchet' face. Difficulty in eating, speaking and swallowing is likely. Severe malocclusion is usual, with expanded arches and labioversion and buccoversion of the teeth producing multiple diastemas. Mandibular dislocation and fracture may occur, presumably indicating some degree of bone weakness. The disease is slowly progressive but patients should not be denied appropriate orthodontic care.

Hemifacial Spasm

This may occur without obvious cause or may result from a tumour at the cerebello-pontine angle. The name is self-explanatory and describes the nature of the disorder.

Oral Complaints in Patients Receiving Phenothiazine Derivatives

Phenothiazine derivatives are widely used as major tranquillizers and to control nausea and vomiting. They act on the extrapyramidal areas of the central nervous system, affecting the basal ganglia. Transient abnormalities of muscle tone have been reported in patients receiving these drugs and the reaction may fail to subside after withdrawal of the drug. Complaints such as 'my tongue wanted to stick itself out and my jaws wanted to rub my gums together', 'my tongue sticks to the roof of my mouth', and 'when I swallow all the muscles tighten up', have been reported. Pain and trismus may occur and there may be extreme lateral deviation of the mandible with spontaneous dislocation of it. In extreme cases, there is rigidity and tremor of the whole body and spasm of many muscles, including those of the larynx.

The patient may seek advice from a physician or a dentist and the diagnosis may be very difficult. Careful exclusion of other disease is required.

Mouthing

Elderly, edentulous patients often unconsciously undertake repetitive chewing and licking movements which lead to difficulty in the provision of satisfactory dentures, excoriation of the lips and noisy clicking sounds which disturb nearby patients and relatives. The movements encourage rocking and mobility of the dentures so that these patients may complain of painful mouths due to denture irritation. Frequently, they are more comfortable without dentures. Dentures are sometimes worn only at mealtimes, although these elderly patients may have difficulty with mastication and may complain that their food 'gets mixed up' with their dentures. Mouthing movements are inhibited by eye closure, a touch on the face or local anaesthetic application to the mouth, and have been ascribed to degenerative changes in the cerebellum.

Inherited Patterns of Movement

Hereditary chin trembling, appearing at birth or soon after, is a rare abnormality which may be associated with tongue-biting during sleep. There is no information as to the precise neurological fault involved.

Many people have the ability to roll up the lateral edges of the protruded tongue while depressing its central portion. This ability, described as tongue rolling, is strongly influenced by hereditary factors and is not usually associated with any other abnormality.

FURTHER READING

Chamberlain, E. N. & Ogilvie, C. (1967) Chapters 9 and 10 in *Symptoms and Signs in Clinical Medicine.* Bristol: John Wright & Sons.
Passmore, R. & Robson, J. S. (Eds.) (1974) Chapter 34 in *A Companion to Medical Studies,* Volume 3. Oxford: Blackwell.

Mental Disease

INTRODUCTION

This chapter provides an abbreviated classification of psychiatric disease and definitions of the more common disturbances. These are necessarily incomplete and the reader is referred to textbooks of psychiatric medicine for comprehensive coverage of the subject. The diagnosis and treatment of psychiatric disease is outside the scope of dentistry and the dentist should avoid any temptation to attempt this. The dentist's function is to exclude dental disease as a cause of symptoms and to ensure that patients with suspected psychiatric disease receive help from a physician. In suggesting such referral the dentist should avoid any implication of mental disorder in conversation with the patient, but he must inform the physician of those signs and symptoms which have led him to suspect the presence of a psychiatric disorder. The dentist will often treat patients who have known mental disturbance and he must have time and under-standing for these patients who may benefit from the simple process of receiving dental care in a sympathetic and well-ordered environment.

The student should realize that it is normal to be sad, or jolly, withdrawn, or tense, depressed or compulsive under some circumstances and to a degree. He may recognize aspects of his own character in the accounts which follow and this is to be expected. Nevertheless, psychiatric complaints are commonplace, and about 10 per cent of the population of the United Kingdom seek medical assistance for these each year. Treatment of these diseases is often highly successful, and it is tragic if patients fail to seek, or are denied, such treatment.

In addition, the dentist must have information about the drugs which a patient who has psychiatric disease is receiving. He must be aware of the possible interactions between the drugs used in the treatment of mental disorders and the drugs he is likely to use in dentistry. The reader is referred to textbooks of pharmacology for information on this subject.

CLASSIFICATION OF MENTAL ILLNESS

1. Neurosis
2. Depression
3. Personality disorders
4. Schizophrenia
5. Organic brain disease
6. Psychosomatic disorders
7. Transient situational disturbances
8. Behaviour disorders of childhood and adolescence
9. Mental retardation.

Neurosis

The term 'neurosis' describes a chronic disorder often associated with anxiety and minor mood disturbance. The patient does not experience hallucinations or delusions and maintains contact with reality, having an awareness of the illness and being able to integrate in society. In contrast, the term 'psychosis' often describes more severe mental illness wherein there is a loss of contact with reality. There are many variations of neurosis. The following examples are considered:

Anxiety neurosis
Phobic neurosis
Hysterical neurosis
Obsessional compulsive neurosis
Hypochondriacal neurosis

Anxiety Neurosis (Free Floating Anxiety)

The patient is conscious of anxiety which is accompanied by restlessness, muscular tension, tremor and excessive sweating. The anxiety may be constant or periodic and may be precipitated by mild stresses or appear without obvious cause. Such patients may complain of pain of the facial pain dysfunction syndrome type as a manifestation of their anxiety or as aggravated by their neurotic tendency.

Phobic Neurosis (Focal Anxiety)

The patient's disease consists of a fear of some object or situation such as open or closed spaces, animals or certain situations. In treating patients with phobias, the dentist should avoid the particular phobic object or situation as the patient may desire. It is foolish to imagine that a dentist's strong personality will overcome the patient's phobia during the short course of a dental treatment session.

Hysterical Neurosis

In the conversion type of hysterical neurosis, the patient 'converts' an anxiety to a physical symptom with consequent relief from the anxiety. Areas of anaesthesia, perhaps affecting the face and lacking any relationship to nerve distribution, or unexpected paralysis may occur, and patients may also demonstrate abnormal movements such as twitching. The patient may appear indifferent to the symptom, perhaps smiling as it is discussed. Sometimes it is apparent that the patient gains from the 'illness' because it provides an escape from the factor causing the anxiety. Such gain may perpetuate the situation.

Obsessional Compulsive Neurosis

The patient has a recurring unwanted thought or irresistible impulse to perform certain acts. The possibilities are endless. For example, a patient may wash his hands for several minutes after using a public lavatory. Then, turning off the water, he feels the necessity to wash again because his hand has touched the tap, and then again after touching the door, and again as he touches the hand rail outside, and so on.

Hypochondriacal Neurosis

Patients with this form of neurosis are preoccupied with health and may have many symptoms. Negative results on investigation provide no reassurance, and the patient is likely to believe that something has been missed. The dentist must avoid needlessly repeated investigations and unnecessary treatment in such cases.

Depression

The classification of depression is a matter of controversy and continuing dialogue among psychiatrists. It is more important that the dentist should have a clear idea of the clinical features of depression than become involved in this discussion, since his duty is to be aware of the existence of this illness and refer those patients who show evidence of it to a physician for proper diagnosis and treatment.

In depression, there is a change of mood so that sadness begins to dominate the patient's outlook. This sadness may be experienced as gloom, fearfulness, despair or self-criticism, and as the illness worsens it is not relieved by reassurance which only serves to irritate and annoy. Eventually, the patient becomes apathetic and convinced of an impending dreadful doom awaiting him and, perhaps, those around him. Onlookers are aware of physical and mental dullness as the patient's thought processes and activity are progressively reduced and of a deterioration in his clothing and personal cleanliness. The self-criticism is common and continued, and the patient blames himself for real or imagined faults. He is fearful in respect of minor symptoms, such as furred tongue or dry mouth, and may become convinced that he is suffering from some serious illness. The dentist who is presented with a catalogue of minor complaints may fail to identify the underlying depression. Sleep disturbances and loss of energy and appetite are likely. Patients may speak of suicide, and suicide or attempted suicide is an important complication of depression. The dentist should not ignore any suggestion of this nature but should ensure that the patient receives immediate care from a physician.

Patients with depression may develop oral disease through lack of care. Thus, one patient came to a dentist complaining of a painful mouth. A diagnosis of vitamin deficiency was made and the patient's diet was found to be inadequate. Further probing revealed the death of a much-loved relative nine months before and profound depression since. The patient's depression yielded to appropriate medical care and the diet improved. The stomatitis was cured without further treatment.

Other patients with depression may exaggerate mild or insignificant symptoms in their desire for help. The dentist should be aware that symptoms such as facial pain or burning tongue may represent such a cry for help. The dentist's obligation is to exclude dental causes of pain and to arrange a consultation with the patient's physician if depression is suspected.

Personality Disorders

These are life-long disorders which demonstrate themselves in the behaviour of individuals as they follow basic instincts, adjust to society, and relate with other individuals. In any one of these situations the behaviour may be unacceptable in a society which regards itself as civilized. There are many varieties of personality disorder, and inadequate and hysterical personalities may be considered as examples.

Inadequate Personality

The individual with an inadequate personality finds difficulty in coping with life. These patients are ineffectual, easily influenced and often unemployed because they cannot fulfil the requirements of any job. Frequently they are charming and as harmless as they are helpless; being more fitted to the embracing care of the village community of a bygone age than to the harsh demands of the contemporary urban society. Such patients provide a considerable burden on the whole range of welfare services, and the dentist called to treat them may find the task time-consuming and frustrating. Nevertheless, dental care should be provided and the dentist may find it helpful to discuss the case with the patient's physician.

Hysterical Personality

People with a hysterical personality remain emotionally immature throughout life. They are self-centred and demanding in a childish fashion, and are apt to 'create a scene' if some petty desire is frustrated. They are shallow in their relationships with others so that situations such as marriage may not survive the minor difficulties which many couples experience. This shallowness may be apparent in their relationships with the dentist, who should beware of the tendency to flirt which is often part of the hysterical personality. The patient lacks awareness of the implications of such flirting. Such patients demand much, but when they are unable to fulfil their share of the dental care programme they are likely to ascribe blame to the dentist when this fails to achieve the desired results. Such patients may manifest the type of hysterical conversion reaction described elsewhere, although others with quite normal personalities may also show this disorder under conditions of severe stress.

Paranoid Personality

Paranoid states are characterized by a feeling of persecution, by the belief that individuals singly or in groups are intent on harming the affected person. Mild paranoid tendencies are commonplace and many people experience these. A few exhibit an excessive suspiciousness of others throughout life. Although never considered mentally ill, such people are described as having a paranoid personality.

Classical paranoia, an extreme form of the disorder unaccompanied by other symptoms, is rare. Paranoid ideas may also occur in psychosis due to organic brain disease, in schizophrenia and in the depressive illnesses.

Oral manifestations are unlikely, although the dentist may join others as seeming to be hostile and threatening in the patient's view of life.

Schizophrenia

This term refers to a group of disorders characterized by disturbances of thought, mood and behaviour. The patient appears to lack emotion or to show inappropriate emotion, perhaps to conceal innermost thoughts from the hostility he imagines around him. In conversation, changes of topic occur without reason or explanation. Fantasy and day-dreaming substitute for reality and the patient's thinking is inward and self-centred. His jokes refer to some secret world and are understood only by himself. The patient will want and not want the same object or objective at the same time. Delusions, hallucinations and a tendency to refer everything, including the conversations and actions of others, to himself may occur. Communication with the patient becomes increasingly difficult, although his intellectual function may be maintained.

The dentist is likely to find that such patients require time and very much tact. They may imagine him to be hostile and they may suspect that quite normal surgery activities are arranged to harm them. Conversation, case-history taking and explanations in respect of treatment may be difficult, or not really meaningful in the ordinary sense, when the patient flits from subject to subject and answer to answer. Occasionally, the patient's hallucinations affect the mouth. For example, one patient complained of pink bubbles which issued from his gums and filled the mouth, then, overflowing, filled the room and floated through the window into the valley: all this was described in fine detail by the patient who was terrified by the 'event'. The dentist should treat such patients in consultation with their physician. Treatment may be delayed during exacerbations of the patient's illness and should always be in a calm surgery with no interruptions. Those involved in the treatment should be visible to the patient and conversation other than with the patient should be discouraged. The amount and extent of treatment will depend on the patient's attitude but should be restricted to a minimum if the patient is markedly disturbed.

Organic Brain Disease

Brain damage caused by infections such as syphilis, intoxications as in alcoholism, trauma, circulatory deficiency, epilepsy, metabolic and nutritional abnormalities, intracranial neoplasms, degenerative processes, and senility, may produce a variety of symptoms. These include lack of awareness of time, place or person, memory loss (particularly for recent events), intellectual impairment, character change showing as impaired judgement and a tendency to social error, atypical reactions such as laughing or crying at some trivial incident, illusions, delusions and hallucinations. The physician must recognize when organic brain disease is causing symptoms such as those described above, since failure to do so results in failure to treat the underlying disease and this may sometimes have a tragic outcome. The dentist may be surprised by a change in character of an old patient; one previously intelligent and witty may become dull and foolish in minor actions. Or the dentist may be exasperated by a patient's forgetfulness in respect of appointments and instructions, particularly in someone previously regarded as a model patient. Consultation with the patient's physician will provide information as to the patient's underlying disease or, rarely, the observations of the dentist may serve to alert the physician to the possibility of organic brain disease, as stated above.

Psychosomatic Disorders

These are also often referred to as psychophysiological disorders, and they are diseases actually produced or aggravated by emotional disturbances. The symptoms are not symbolical representations of these disturbances, as in the neuroses. Scientific proof of emotional involvement in these diseases is often lacking and every effort should be made to exclude actual organic disease.

The mouth has an important involvement in the mother—child relationship and with the vital intake or rejection of food. It is involved in the show of aggression and in sexual play. So it is not surprising that emotional disturbance may cause oral symptoms. Bruxism which causes pain or damage to the dentition, the temporo-mandibular joint pain dysfunction syndrome, atypical facial pain, glossodynia, and xerostomia may, on occasion, represent psychosomatic disorders. Often, proof of such an aetiology is lacking and the clinician reaches a diagnosis by a process of exclusion and an understanding of the patient's psyche. The dentist can play an important role in the first leg of diagnosis, that is, in the exclusion of dental disease, but the dentist's surgery is not the best place for proper psychiatric evaluation nor is the dentist competent in this role.

Transient Situational Disorders

These may present as anxiety or depression and a sense of inability to cope with a situation. Insomnia and fatigue are common. There are many causes of such disorders; for example, the executive faced with increased responsibility, or the housewife faced with total responsibility for the home and family because of her husband's death, absence or illness. The patient may overemphasize some oral complaint or complain of headache due to muscle tension.

Behaviour Disorders of Childhood and Adolescence

There are many varieties of behaviour disorder and these are of interest to the dentist since failure to recognize them may lead him to reject a child or adolescent as a 'bad patient', thus further aggravating the disorder. The dentist who seeks guidance from the child's physician before treating the difficult child and who pays due attention to the behaviour disorder may obtain regard and trust from a young person who too often has found difficulty in trusting others.

Some children are excessively active, their restlessness causing constant disruption in classroom or family. Such hyperactivity may indicate brain damage or may occur from other causes. Other children, excessively shy and full of anxiety, may have suffered deprivation or suppression in their family situation.

Mental Retardation

This is a state of arrested, imperfect or subnormal intellectual ability which appears in childhood and interferes with learning and with adaptation to the environment and to social situations. Mental retardation has many causes and these are listed below, with a single illustrative example of each:

Infections — rubella in the first trimester of pregnancy.
Intoxications — high serum bilirubin due to rhesus incompatibility.
Trauma — brain injury during delivery.
Disorders of metabolism and nutrition — cretinism.
New growths — neurofibromatosis.
Congenital cerebral defects and chromosomal disorders — mongolism.
Severe deprivation — blindness and deafness.

There are no special oral manifestations of mental retardation, although the tongue is described as large in mongolism and in cretinism, and there is a tendency to salivate. However, retarded children and adults require dental care as do other patients, and the dentist treating such patients with tact and understanding will be rewarded with such trust and affection as the patient is capable of. Mental retardation receives attention in some textbooks of paedodontics and in specialist works.

CONCLUSIONS

The dentist must avoid diagnosis of mental illness, since this is outside his area of competence. He should always ensure that his first duty is to exclude dental causes for symptoms, although an awareness of the spectrum of mental disorder may provide clues in the diagnosis of some patients. Above all, the dentist should be aware of those situations where depression may place a patient in serious risk of suicide and ensure that such patients are provided with medical assistance as a matter of priority.

FURTHER READING

Bond, M. R. (1978) *Understanding People.* Edinburgh: Churchill Livingstone.
Harris, M. (1974) Psychogenic aspects of facial pain. *British Dental Journal,* **136,** 199—202.
Passmore, R. & Robson, J. S. (Eds.) (1974) Chapter 35 in *A Companion to Medical Studies,* Volume 3. Oxford: Blackwell.

part 7

DISEASE OF THE
LYMPHORETICULAR SYSTEM

chapter 23

Cervicofacial Lymphadenopathy

Local Infection
General Infection
Other Diseases
Neoplasms
The Approach to Diagnosis of Cervical Lymphadenopathy

The lymph nodes have two major functions: first, they are concerned with the inter-ception and removal of abnormal or foreign material in the lymph draining to them and, second, they have an important role in the production of the immune response. The lymphatic system of the head and neck region is illustrated diagrammatically in Figure 23.1. As at least 25 per cent of the lymph glands in the body are situated in the head and neck region, it is not surprising that the cervicofacial lymph glands are important markers of disease states.

Disease affecting the cervicofacial lymph glands may be classified on an aetiological basis as due to acute or chronic infection, neoplasms or connective tissue disease (Table 23.1).

The oral manifestations of many of the conditions listed in Table 23.1 are described elsewhere in this book but those which are not will now be considered.

LOCAL INFECTION

By far the commonest local cause of cervical lymph gland enlargement is infection which may be due to any of a large number of different viruses (for example, herpes simplex, coxsackie) which affect the oropharyngeal and upper respiratory regions.

Pyogenic bacterial infections, from infected teeth, mucosa, scalp, ears and tonsils are also common. Treatment consists of controlling the infection and eradicating the cause. The prescribing of antibiotics without a careful follow-up investigation to identify and treat the source of the infection is to be deprecated.

Submandibular and cervical lymph nodes can be infected with atypical mycobacteria and this is an important cause of cervical lymphadenitis in children. Atypical

261

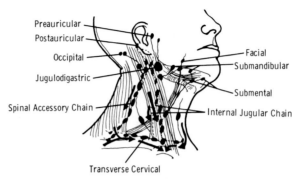

Figure 23.1. The lymphatic system of the head and neck region.

mycobacteria are more resistant to chemotherapeutic agents than the tubercle bacilli and in persistent cases surgery is the treatment of choice.

Infection with *Mycobacterium tuberculosis* occurs much less commonly now but causes chronic soft enlargement of the cervical glands following tonsillar infection. The Mantoux test is always strongly positive. Indurated cervical glands usually accompany the primary chancre of lip or tongue which occurs in syphilis.

Cat scratch disease occurs rarely and is thought to be due to chlamydiae which act by gaining entrance through a superficial skin lesion and producing a cervical lymphadenopathy. There is no curative treatment for this condition which lasts for a period of some weeks to several months.

Table 23.1. *Classification of disease affecting the cervicofacial lymph glands.*

Infections:	Pyogenic infection
	Atypical mycobacteria
	T.B.; Syphilis
	Cat scratch fever
	Infectious mononucleosis (glandular fever)
	German measles (rubella)
	Toxoplasmosis
Other diseases:	Sarcoidosis
	Connective tissue disease (rheumatoid arthritis; systemic lupus erythematosus)
	Lipid storage disease (histiocytosis)
Neoplasms:	Lymphomas
	Leukaemias
	Metastases from other malignant neoplasms

GENERAL INFECTION

Infectious mononucleosis (glandular fever) is thought to be due to infection with the Epstein—Barr virus. It occurs in small epidemics and principally affects young adults. It is characterized by tender swollen cervical lymph glands, low-grade fever which lasts from one to three weeks, and the presence of abnormal lymphoid cells in the blood. The posterior cervical lymph glands are usually affected first. Prominent clinical features are malaise, headache, skin rash and sore throat. The disease is diagnosed by a positive monospot screening test followed by the Paul—Bunnell haemagglutination test. There is also a raised ESR, lymphocytosis and the presence of atypical lymphocytes in the blood. The course of the disease is variable, with a two- to ten-week duration, and is seldom fatal. The oral manifestations of infectious mononucleosis are considered in Chapter 4.

In German measles (rubella) mild constitutional symptoms are accompanied by nasal catarrh and conjunctivitis. The illness is usually over in two to three days. There is usually a history of previous contact or knowledge of an epidemic. Early clinical manifestations are some stiffness of the neck and the development of slightly tender and enlarged posterior cervical lymph glands. The rash usually appears on the second day and is often the first indication of the disease. It consists of thick macules which appear first behind the ears and on the forehead, and then spread to involve the trunk and the limbs. There may be more generalized enlargement of the cervical lymph glands in addition to the sub-occipital group.

Histoplasmosis is a rare condition affecting lymph glands. It presents as a localized respiratory infection but may also cause an acute generalized involvement of lymph nodes, spleen, bone marrow and liver by the organism *Histoplasma capsulatum*. This infection results in granulomatous foci in the affected tissues which heal with calcification. The clinical manifestations can simulate tuberculosis.

Infection with the protozoon *Toxoplasma gondii* may occur anywhere in the world but is more common in warm or moist than in cold or dry climates. It may occur at any age but most often occurs in young adults and often presents as painless localized or generalized lymphadenopathy. Other organs — lungs, heart and skeletal muscle — may be affected. The protozoon exists in two forms: the proliferative and the cystic, and many animals carry the organism in their excreta, including saliva. A rising titre of antibody can be demonstrated by the dye exclusion test. Antiprotozoal drugs such as pyrimethamine with sulphonamides may be used in treatment but pyrimethamine has toxic side-effects.

OTHER DISEASES

Sarcoidosis

Enlargement of lymph glands is a common manifestation of sarcoidosis and the cervical glands are commonly involved. Other clinical features are mild fever, malaise, loss of weight, arthritis, iritis and erythema nodosum. Lung involvement is common and on chest x-ray the hilar lymph glands are usually enlarged. Oral mucosal involvement is rare but salivary glands are often affected (see Chapter 14).

Blood examinations are helpful. There is increased ESR. In addition, leucopenia, eosinophilia, thrombocytopenia, hyperproteinaemia and hypercalcaemia may occur. The elevated serum proteins are due to elevated alpha-2, beta and gamma globulins.

There is a deficiency in the delayed type cutaneous sensitivity. Patients with sarcoid usually have the following skin tests:

1. Kveim test. The Kveim antigen is a 10 per cent suspension of proved sarcoid tissue in normal saline solution. The test is performed by the intradermal injection of 0.2 ml Kveim antigen in the forearm. After six weeks the site (which has to be accurately marked) is excised and the typical sarcoid granuloma signifies a positive Kveim reaction.
2. Mantoux test. The majority of patients with sarcoid are negative tuberculin reactors or become positive reactors only at high concentrations.

Biopsy of a cutaneous sarcoid lesion or an enlarged lymph node is a more rapid method of confirming the diagnosis. As lymph gland involvement is common, a lymph gland biopsy may also be carried out in suspected cases even when lymph gland enlargement is not present. The scalene node situated in the cervical region is usually selected. The typical histological appearances include an epithelioid cell follicle with central Langhans' type giant cells without caseation or tubercle bacilli. The giant cells may contain asteroid inclusion bodies, known as Schaumann's bodies, which contain calcium.

Connective Tissue Disease

In both rheumatoid arthritis and in systemic lupus erythematosus a mild to moderate lymph gland enlargement may occur.

Lipid Storage Diseases or Histiocytosis

These include three conditions which are characterized by histcytic proliferation and replacement of bone marrow and bone as well as infiltration of other tissues, including lymph glands. These conditions are eosinophilic granuloma of bone, which occurs in adults, Hand—Schüller—Christian disease, which usually affects children, and Letterer—Siwe disease, in infants. These conditions are of unknown aetiology. The accumulation of lipids follows the proliferation of histiocytes. There is no lipidaemia or known abnormality of lipid metabolism. Although each condition has a variable prognosis, from eosinophilic granuloma which is benign to Letterer—Siwe disease which is lethal, and affects different age groups, it would appear that they are possibly related with regard to aetiology and pathogenesis.

The first oral manifestation of the disease may be loosening of teeth for no apparent reason. Radiographs will show clearly demarcated areas of radiolucency where the bone is involved. Diagnosis will be confirmed by biopsy of an affected area of oral tissue or cervical lymph gland.

NEOPLASMS

The Lymphomas

The exact histogenesis of these tumours is doubtful but there is good evidence that many of them originate from the lymphoid series of cells. As a group they vary greatly in prognosis from causing death in a matter of weeks to running a chronic course. They can arise in any tissue but most commonly arise in lymph glands, spleen, bone marrow, liver skin and gastrointestinal tract. It is not possible to draw a sharp line of demarcation between the leukaemias and lymphoma.

The classification of lymphomas has not yet reached a rational stage. It is generally agreed that Hodgkin's disease is a distinct entity. The remaining or non-Hodgkin's lymphomas can be grouped into follicular lymphomas and diffuse lymphomas, each of which may be of low or high grade malignancy. Most of these non-Hodgkin's lymphomas are thought to be of B-lymphocyte lineage except for some of the diffuse or non-follicular high-grade-malignancy type, some of which are of T-cell origin.

Hodgkin's Disease

The disease can occur at any age with peaks in early and late adult life. The usual presenting feature is progressive painless enlargement of lymph nodes, cervical, inguinal or axillary. Constitutional symptoms, low-grade fever which sometimes exhibits a periodic pattern (Pel—Ebstein fever), anaemia and leucocytosis occur. Cell-mediated immunity is impaired and patients are prone to infections by opportunistic organisms such as herpes zoster, fungae and tubercle bacilli. The enlarged lymph nodes are discrete and rubbery (Figure 23.2).

The prognosis varies from death in a few months to good health for many years even without treatment. Diagnosis and treatment are related to the histological pattern observed on biopsy of an affected lymph node. The extent of the disease is critical for assessing the prognosis and in planning therapy. A process of staging, from involvement of one node to widespread involvement of one or more non-lymphoid tissues, is used and, along with the histological typing, will determine the choice of treatment from radiotherapy or systemic chemotherapy.

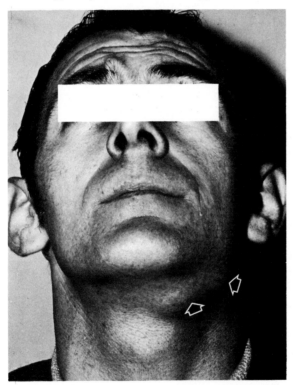

Figure 23.2. Hodgkin's disease presenting as painless enlargement of L submandibular glands. On palpation, the glands were of 'rubbery' texture.

Other Lymphomas or Non-Hodgkin's Lymphomas

These include the following:

Follicular lymphoma. This occurs principally in old people. Lymph glands are mainly involved. Although follicular lymphoma is generally of low grade malignancy initially, it can change from an initial slow growth to a more aggressive type. Diagnosis is made on the histological appearance of numerous follicular structures which resemble normal reactive germinal centres but contain abnormal cells.

Diffuse lymphoma. Most tumours in this group are widely disseminated. Generalized lymphadenopathy and hepatosplenomegaly are present and the enlarged nodes may cause pressure effects. Those of low-grade malignancy are usually sensitive to chemotherapeutic agents, such as chlorambucil, and the prognosis is generally good. The other diffuse lymphomas, which are of high-grade malignancy, are locally destructive and metastasize by lymphatics or blood to distant sites. They require staging and typing, as do other lymphomas, before treatment can be planned. Typing is more difficult in these cases because the lymphomas are mostly blast cells. The lympho-blastic lymphomas are the commonest lymphomas of childhood and adolescence, except for Hodgkin's disease. These tumours may be of T-cell origin and may progress to acute lymphoblastic leukaemia.

Burkitt's lymphoma. A special variant of lymphoma is Burkitt's lymphoma which is a lymphosarcoma occurring extensively in certain humid regions of Central and West Africa. It particularly affects children up to the age of 15 years and commonly presents as jaw enlargement, the maxilla being more commonly affected than the mandible. Teeth in the area of the swelling become loose. Other tissues affected are the lymph nodes, ovaries and kidneys. The most exciting aspect of this condition is the growing evidence that it is caused by the Epstein—Barr virus. Patients develop immune responses to both the virus and tumour-specific antigens. Those individuals with good immune responses derive remarkable benefit from tumour chemotherapy and it is suggested that the chemotherapy lessens the vitality of the tumour cells and allows the immune response to control them.

As has been mentioned above, the·Epstein—Barr virus has also been implicated in glandular fever, another disease which affects lymphoid tissue. It has been suggested that Burkitt's lymphoma and glandular fever are different manifestations of infection with the same virus.

A positive relationship has also been noted between the incidence, in the same district, of Burkitt's lymphoma and malaria. It has been suggested that the antigen—antibody complexes from the malarial attack block cell-mediated response against the Epstein—Barr virus, with resultant persistence of the virus and tumour formation.

Leukaemias. The leukaemias are considered as a group in Chapter 8.

Metastases from Other Neoplasms

Lymphatic spread of other malignant neoplasms, especially carcinoma, is very common. Cervical gland metastases occur from squamous cell carcinoma of the oral mucosa and from carcinoma of other parts of the head and neck region. It may also occur from more distant primary sites, such as bronchi, thyroid, breast, oesophagus, stomach or pancreas. Although most sarcomas spread via the blood, lymph node involvement may occur in the case of rhabdomyosarcoma and sarcomas of synovial origin.

THE APPROACH TO DIAGNOSIS OF CERVICAL LYMPHADENOPATHY

The patient who presents with swelling of the cervical lymph glands should have a complete history taken. This should include the following questions:

1. What is the duration of the enlargement?
2. Was the enlargement accompanied by pain?
3. Has enlargement been progressive or has it varied in size?
4. When enlargement occurred, did the patient have any constitutional upsets, such as fever or any other symptoms or signs?
5. Has the enlargement been associated with any pain or swelling around the oral region?

On examining the patient it is important to follow the method described in Chapter 2. The neck should be fully exposed and a systematic approach should be used, with examination, in turn, of the occipital, mastoid, parotid, submental, submandibular and upper and lower cervical glands. It may be difficult to distinguish between sub-mandibular salivary glands and submandibular lymph glands but bimanual examination, with one finger on the floor of the mouth, may be helpful. The tonsils should also be examined in the course of full intra-oral examination. The skin and common less-accessible sites of infection in the head and neck region, such as scalp and ears, should also be carefully examined and, where indicated, the patient may be referred for a full ear, nose and throat examination. In general, lymph glands associated with acute infections are enlarged, tender or painful, soft and discrete. In chronic infections, the lymph nodes are less painful or painless and soft-to-firm in nature. Secondary metastases of carcinoma in lymph glands produces hard glands which may be attached to underlying tissues. The glands in Hodgkin's disease and other lymphomas are described as rubbery-to-firm in character.

In every case where cervical lymph gland enlargement is found and where there is no obvious local cause, other sites of the reticulo-endothelial system should be examined, including other accessible lymph glands, such as the axillary and inguinal, as well as the liver and the spleen. A chest radiograph will demonstrate enlargement of the hilar lymph glands if they are involved.

After a full history and physical examination it may be necessary to proceed to further investigations, such as blood examination, radiological examination (including sialography), microbiological examination or biopsy.

part 8

RESEARCH

chapter 24

Clinical Research in Oral Medicine

Introduction
Example of Analysis of a Therapeutic Trial

INTRODUCTION

The discipline of oral medicine is still in its infancy compared with other clinical specialties and, as such, a vast amount of information is required about the aetiology, diagnosis and treatment of conditions which affect the mouth and perioral tissues. The literature continues to describe new diseases which occur in the mouth, together with their associations with lesions elsewhere in the body. It is essential, therefore, that departments of oral medicine be deeply involved in research and develop a scientific approach to all aspects of the subject. It is no longer acceptable to conduct programmes of management or prescribe treatments unless these have been critically examined and subjected to therapeutic trials.

The first basic essential in any clinical research project is to define, lucidly and precisely, the aim of the research. At the same time, the feasibility of carrying out this project with human beings must be examined and the ethics of the situation considered. A guideline on ethics in human research is given in the Declaration of Helsinki: the basis of this document is that clinical research should be conducted by suitably qualified individuals and should conform to accepted scientific and moral principles. Prior to conducting any research on humans the full text of this declaration should be consulted.

It is now customary to have an Ethics Committee in hospitals wherein research is liable to be conducted. This usually consists of senior members of staff as well as interested lay persons and its purpose is to examine all clinical research projects prior to their initiation. Once a project has been approved by such a group, any research procedures must be clearly explained to patients and no pressure should be placed upon them to participate. If the patient agrees to take part this is termed *informed consent*. Patients are entitled to refuse to participate in a research project and have the right to receive conventional management.

Therapeutic trials of drugs from commercial companies come under the additional surveillance of the Committee for Safety of Drugs in Medicine (in Britain) or the Food and Drugs Administration (in the U.S.A.).

Clinical research may be conducted in various areas: it may be directed towards identifying the aetiology of the disorder, discovering the best method of diagnosing the disease, or assessing current treatment and investigating new methods of treatment. Each objective requires that different criteria be answered, and a suitable approach should be generated for each.

The following general basic approach should be adopted. The aim of the research programme should be stated and a protocol developed to summarize the entire procedure in the order that it is to be carried out. At this stage the various possible answers should be capable of interpretation and statistical analysis. If there is the least doubt at this initial, critical point then the assistance of a statistician should be sought. There is little point in accumulating data which may be uninterpretable or ambiguous.

Studies can be retrospective or prospective. While strict conditions and a protocol can be developed for a prospective study these criteria are often not available when findings are to be examined retrospectively. Retrospective studies are sometimes necessary, however, as they may be the only way of amassing sufficient information to be of use in the immediate future. It is not always practical to envisage what data may be relevant in the future and the only safeguard is to ensure that whatever information is obtained is clearly set out in case notes. As a means of facilitating future retrospective analyses, many clinical departments are developing systems, either manual or computerized, of categorizing diseases. Such disease indices list all cases with the same diagnosis and permit rapid retrieval of information without anyone having to scrutinize every case note in the hospital files. The two such systems most commonly used are (a) International Classification of Disease and (b) Systematic Nomenclature of Pathology.

In order to obtain some idea of the prevalence and gravity of any particular disease the mortality figures can be examined. These date back for a considerable period in most countries and also reveal how disease patterns change with time. Unfortunately, the data are of limited value in oral diseases as so many are either not fatal or else not previously recognized.

Cross-sectional studies of the population can be carried out to obtain the prevalence of a particular disorder at any one time. Correlations can be made regarding age, sex, environment and occupation. Hence it may be possible to make some deductions about aetiology.

Specific groups can be selected and, matched against a suitable control group, they can be examined in a temporal or longitudinal manner, thus also providing data about the incidence or occurrence of new cases. This is of value when examining potential aetiological factors or the effect of preventive measures.

The selection of individuals for inclusion in a test sample should be made in a random manner: it is often impractical to include the entire population possessing certain parameters and therefore a representative sample must be selected. This is readily accomplished by allocating a number to each member of the entire population and then selecting a series of numbers at random, using standard tables of random numbers.

When designing a trial it may be desirable either to examine a control group of individuals who do not have the disorder, or to treat patients who have the disease with an inert preparation (placebo). Under these circumstances, the selection of controls is based upon matching for age and sex in addition to any other potentially relevant criteria.

The size of a sample requires consideration. It has to be a balance between a number which is eventually capable of statistical analysis while, at the same time, must not contain a greater number of individuals than can be efficiently handled: unmanageable numbers lead to mistakes and poor documentation.

Trials may be conducted in several phases. It is customary to run an initial pilot study with a small number of people prior to proceeding with a large-scale investigation. Any obvious trend or side-effects will emerge at this early stage.

Therapeutic trials may be designed in several ways. Patients can be split into two comparable groups, one group being given an active form of therapy and the other nothing or, preferably, a placebo. Alternatively, in a disorder which is almost continuous, such as many cases of recurrent aphthae, it is possible to use the same group as their own controls by giving half the active preparation followed by the placebo, and the remaining half the placebo followed by the active preparation. When the patients do not know if the treatment is active or a placebo it is termed a 'single-blind trial'. It is possible in some instances that the clinician may influence the subjective response from patients and many trials are therefore conducted with neither the clinician nor the patient knowing what the active preparation is: this is termed a 'double-blind trial'. The code is revealed only upon completion of the trial.

The duration of a study also merits consideration. The longer it runs the more accurate will be the information derived from it but there will be patient losses as well as unnecessary expense and effort. A compromise period should be reached which will be adequate for any significant trend to be detected.

When the period of study is complete, the data are collected and analysed statistically. A discussion of the many techniques of statistics is beyond the scope of this book and the reader is referred to specialized texts.

Essentially, an attempt is made to establish whether the findings could have occurred by chance and the probability of this happening. At the outset the assumption is tentatively made that there is no difference between the different groups under scrutiny. This assumption, termed the 'null hypothesis', is then tested with the data. Should it be wrong for the particular data the findings are significant and unlikely to have arisen by chance.

A probability always exists that a particular finding is a coincidence and occurred by chance, be it one chance in ten or one in a million. It is customary to state the probability of any event happening by chance. A value below 5 per cent ($P<0.05$) is accepted as significant in biological science, and a value below 1 per cent ($P<0.01$) as highly significant.

When the information has been statistically analysed the findings must be interpreted and evaluated. If the investigation was correctly formulated, there should be no ambiguity. If the study has been a therapeutic trial, the benefits of the drug must be balanced against side-effects and these compared to other comparable drugs already in existence. Finally a cost—benefit analysis is undertaken in which the benefit obtained from adopting a certain procedure or form of therapy is weighed against the cost of adopting it.

EXAMPLE OF ANALYSIS OF A THERAPEUTIC TRIAL

Purpose of trial: to evaluate a new drug, X, for the treatment of recurrent aphthae.

Design. Ten patients are used. For the first eight-week period they all maintain a record of the number of ulcers which they have.

They are then given either the drug, X, or else an inert placebo, which is identical in appearance to the drug, for the next eight-week period.

Finally, they are switched around for a final eight weeks, with those who had initially received the placebo now being given the drug and those first given the drug now being given the placebo. In this way each patient not only has a control phase, with no treatment, but also has treatment with a placebo.

Usually, both the drug and placebo are made identical in appearance and neither the patient nor clinician knows what preparation is being used at the time: this double-blind trial eliminates the possibility of the outcome's being influenced subconsciously and the code is revealed only upon completion of the trial.

For the present purpose, no further considerations of the design of such a trial need be considered.

Results

Patient no.	No. of ulcers in first eight weeks	No. of ulcers with placebo	No. of ulcers with drug X
1	24	19	10
2	7	6	2
3	15	17	9
4	32	26	13
5	9	8	8
6	15	17	12
7	27	21	14
8	11	5	6
9	19	13	1
10	30	16	4
Mean	18.90	14.80	7.90
Standard deviation:	8.94	6.80	4.56

By using Student's t test

1. Compare: no treatment with placebo
    $P > 0.2$ (not significant)
2. Compare: no treatment with drug X
    $P < 0.01$ (highly significant)
3. Compare: placebo with drug X
    $P < 0.05$ but > 0.01 (significant)

Conclusion. At first inspection there would appear to be a reduction in the number of ulcers in the patients being given the placebo preparation. However, on closer examination there is a considerable variation between patients in the number of ulcers developing and this is reflected in the relatively high standard deviation. On applying the Student t test, a value for P of greater than 0.2 is obtained and, accordingly, it is concluded that there is no significant difference in the number of ulcers occurring with no treatment or with the placebo.

On the other hand, when drug X is compared with no treatment, a P value of less than 0.01 is obtained and this is a highly significant difference. Likewise, the difference between drug X and the placebo is significant, the P value being less than 0.05.

In trials, it is not uncommon to find a significant response to a placebo preparation and it is important always to compare the active preparation with an inert one.

FURTHER READING

Davies, G. N. (1976) Chapter 58 in Cohen, B. & Kramer, I. R. H. (Eds.) *Scientific Foundations of Dentistry.* London: Heinemann.
Siegel, S. (1956) *Non-parametric Statistics for the Behavioral Sciences.* New York: McGraw-Hill.
Truelove, S. C. (1975) *Medical Surveys and Clinical Trials.* London: Oxford University Press.

Further Investigations — Methods

When a detailed history has been taken and the clinical examination completed, the stage may be reached where there is no single diagnosis but a list of possibilities, that is, a differential diagnosis. At this point it is necessary to conduct further investigations in order to establish the final diagnosis.

It is of the utmost importance that the potential value of any one test be appreciated with regard to its reliability in diagnosing a disorder as well as to the incidence of false-positive and false-negative results. Laboratories may be overwhelmed with requests for numerous investigations which are not really justified. On occasion, samples are sent off by a clinician instead of conducting a proper clinical examination or because he has failed to elaborate a differential diagnosis and he is 'shooting blindly'.

When such an indiscriminating approach to further investigations is adopted, not only is time wasted in examining urgent and relevant cases but substantial costs can be incurred.

The clinician should therefore have a knowledge of what investigations are available but at the same time must realize their limitations and make request for them in a rational manner.

Interpretation of investigations requires a knowledge of the various factors which can produce an abnormal result for any one test. A further complicating factor lies in deciding precisely at which point a result is really abnormal, and there is frequently a grey area of borderline values for any investigation: these can fluctuate between abnormal and borderline or normal and borderline and accordingly may have to be repeated.

Another factor in requesting further investigations is practicality. An ideal oral medicine clinic will be situated in a position where all necessary investigations can be carried out with minimal inconvenience and time expenditure. On the other hand, not all centres have functional oral medicine units and the range of tests may be more limited. The general medical practitioner and general dental practitioner can be even more isolated and they are faced with the problems of transporting samples in appropriate containers to specific laboratories. The alternatives are either to select a probable diagnosis based upon clinical judgement, and treat the disorder accordingly, or else to refer the patient.

With the development of health centres or group practices where both medical and dental practitioners function, it can be anticipated that certain investigative procedures will become more amenable.

The common investigations related to problems in oral medicine will now be discussed.

Haematology

Haemoglobin, mean cell volume (MCV), mean corpuscular haemoglobin (MCH), WBC count and blood film: diagnosis of anaemia and of blood dyscrasias. Indication of a nutritional deficiency where iron, folic acid or vitamin B_{12} is lacking (values can be normal in early stages of deficiency): platelet count for thrombocytopenia.

Corrected whole blood (CWB) folate and serum folate: low in folic acid deficiency. CWB folate is a more accurate index of tissue levels as serum folate fluctuates with recent dietary experience.

Serum vitamin B_{12}: Low value is indicative of vitamin B_{12} deficiency. Not diagnostic of pernicious anaemia specifically.

Schilling test: For diagnosis of pernicious anaemia. This is a functional test of vitamin B_{12} metabolism, using a radioactive isotope.

Marrow: Evidence of iron, folic acid and vitamin B_{12} deficiency. White cell dyscrasias and marrow aplasia.

Coagulation studies: For diagnosis of bleeding tendency, including haemophilia.

Sickle cell anaemia test: Indicative of individuals who have both sickle cell anaemia and the trait. (Also haemoglobin electrophoresis.)

Biochemistry

Serum iron and total iron binding capacity: Lowered iron and raised total iron binding capacity (TIBC), with a saturation under 16 per cent (i.e. $\frac{IRON}{TIBC} \times 100$) indicative of iron deficiency.

Serum ferritin: Lowered in iron deficiency.

Serum calcium, phosphate and alkaline phosphatase: Abnormal in cases of active bone turnover or destruction, e.g. increased parathyroid function or Paget's disease of bone.

Plasma glucose: Raised fasting level in diabetes mellitus along with abnormal glucose tolerance test.

Serum protein and electrophoresis: Abnormalities in chronic inflammation, immune disorders and certain lymphomas.

Urinalysis for glucose: Positive in diabetes mellitus.

Urinalysis for protein: May be positive in SLE.

Faecal fat: Increased in malabsorption.

Faecal occult blood: Indicative of blood loss into alimentary tract, e.g. peptic ulcer, carcinoma, haemorrhoids.

Leucocyte ascorbic acid: Lowered in scurvy.

Immunology

Rheumatoid factor: Indicative of rheumatoid arthritis.

Anti-nuclear factor (ANF): Indicative of systemic lupus erythematosus (SLE).

DNA binding: More specific in diagnosis of SLE.

Salivary duct antibody: Relatively non-specific. Variable interpretation.

IgA reticulin antibody: Suggestive of coeliac disease.

Antibody to intercellular area of spinous cells in stratified squamous epithelium: Suggestive of pemphigus vulgaris (blood group substances having been adsorbed out).

Antibody to basement membrane region of stratified squamous epithelium: Suggestive of pemphigoid.

Direct fluorescent antibody in frozen sections of mucosa or skin: Suggestive of pemphigus, or pemphigoid, according to distribution (as above).

Pathology

Cytology: Not used much and difficult to interpret.

Biopsy (frozen): Very rapid diagnosis (only rarely, where speed is critical and in tissues where distortion of freezing does not make the diagnosis uncertain). Also used for direct fluorescent antibody technique to demonstrate bound immunoglobulins in tissue.

Biopsy (fixed): For conventional histopathological diagnosis. Occasionally, electron microscopy is carried out.

Jejunal biopsy: Diagnostic for coeliac disease.

Labial biopsy of minor salivary glands: Reflects involvement in Sjögren's syndrome.

Microbiology

Smears on to glass slides from lesions and dentures: Essential for detection of candidal hyphae. Gram stain of smear permits tentative comment on organisms within five minutes.

Swab for bacteriology: Culture of organisms, identification and antibiotic sensitivity.

Swab for virology in transport medium: Isolation of viruses, e.g. herpes simplex.

Serum during acute phase and in convalescent phase of viral infection: Rising titre (fourfold) confirms the viral infection.

Paul-Bunnell test: For infectious mononucleosis.

Radiology

Direct views: Various bony disorders.

Tomography: Used to visualize the temporomandibular joints.

Sialography: Infusion injection of aqueous radio-opaque media into ducts of major salivary glands to visualize the morphology of the ductal system.

Barium meal and barium enema: Alimentary lesions in blood loss or malabsorption.

Radionucleotide Scanning (Linear-Scintillation Counter or Gamma Camera)

$^{99}Tc^m$*-as pertechnneate (TcO$_4^-$):* Uptake by salivary glands in functional studies. Possible assistance in tumour identification.

Diphosphoate and ^{18}F: Areas of altered bone metabolism, e.g. Paget's disease and fibrous dysplasia.

^{67}Ga*, Indium and ^{75}Se-Selenomethionine:* Potential malignant tumour detection.

Ultrasonography

Potential use in swellings of head and neck. Information about lesion margins as well as intrinsic consistency.

Detection of Endocrine Disorders

Pituitary: Direct measurement of hormones in blood. Measure serum levels following stimulation or depression. Function of target organs.

Adrenal cortex: Diurnal rhythm in serum cortisol. Synacthen test. Metopyrone inhibition of cortisol synthesis. Urinary 17-hydroxy-steroids. Antibodies to adrenal cortex.

Thyroid: Protein bound iodine. Thyroxine and tri-iodothyronine levels. T_3 uptake. Thyroid antibodies (various). Uptake of radioactive iodine and pertechnetate.

Parathyroid: Serum calcium, phosphorus and alkaline phosphatase. Direct serum parathormone.

Gonads: Urinary 17-hydroxysteroids. Serum levels of oestrogens, progesterone and androgens.

Pancreatic islets (β cells): Urine for glucose. Fasting plasma glucose. Glucose tolerance test. Insulin levels in serum.

appendix 2

Drugs Commonly Used in Oral Medicine

The prescribing of drugs is an important aspect of patient treatment in certain oral disorders. The use of these drugs is referred to in the general text and the reader is referred to standard books on pharmacology and therapeutics for greater detail.

The decision to use any particular drug should be carefully considered and prior to selecting a drug the following questions might be asked (after Herxheimer, 1976):

1. *Need*	Is the drug really needed?	
	What is likely to happen if it is not used?	
2. *Class*	To what class does the drug belong?	
3. *Aim*	What aim is to be achieved with the drug?	
	What disorder of function is to be corrected, or what symptom relieved?	
	When are the treatment effects expected to begin?	
4. *Observations*	What observations should be made to judge whether the aim has been achieved?	
	How should serious unwanted effects be watched for?	
	When should these observations be made, and by whom?	
5. *Route and dosage*	By what route, in what dose, at what intervals and at what times is the drug to be given, and why?	
	Up to what limit is it worth increasing dosage and/or frequency if the response is inadequate?	
6. *Alternatives*	What other drugs could be used instead of this one?	
	Do the drugs differ notably in efficacy or safety?	
	Do their costs differ much?	
7. *Duration*	How long should the drug continue to be used, and how will the decision be made to stop?	
8. *Unwanted effects*	What undesirable effects may occur from the drug?	
	Are they acceptable?	
	What is their approximate frequency?	
	How can they be avoided, or treated if they occur?	
9. *Elimination*	How is the drug eliminated?	
	Will the patient's illness change the usual pattern of distribution and effects of the drug? If yes, how does this affect the dosage?	
10. *Interactions*	Are there any other drugs, foods or activities which the patient should avoid while he is receiving the drug?	
11. *Patient's ideas*	What does the patient believe about the drug?	
	What has he been told about it and what does he remember?	
	Does he need additional information?	
	Will he take the drug?	

(a) *Antibiotics for systemic use in various bacterial infections.*

The selection of a suitable antibiotic ideally should be based upon a microbiological sensitivity report. The following are frequently used and their dosages indicated. The first four, being members of the penicillin group, must be avoided in cases of penicillin allergy.

279

	Adult dose	
Phenoxymethyl penicillin	250 mg	four times daily
Amoxycillin	250 mg	three times daily
Talampicillin	250 mg	three times daily
Flucloxacillin	250—500 mg	four times daily
Co-trimoxazole	2 Tablets	twice daily
Erythromycin	250 mg	four times daily
Oxytetracycline	250 mg	four times daily
Clindamycin	150 mg	four times daily
Cephradine	250 mg	four times daily
Metronidazole	200 mg	three times daily

(b) *Topical antibiotics for bacterial infections around the mouth, e.g. angular cheilitis*

Fusidate Ointment
Chlortetracycline Ointment
Miconazole Cream (also active as anti-fungal)

(c) *Antifungal preparations*

Nystatin Amphotericin } creams and ointment Miconazole	For angular cheilitis, with candidal infection. Also for placing on fitting surface of dentures in denture stomatitis.
Amphotericin Lozenges Nystatin tablets and pessaries }	To be sucked six times daily. For candidal infections.
Nystatin Amphotericin } mixtures or suspension Pimafucin	For children or debilitated patients.

(d) *Antiseptic mouthwashes for use in many forms of oral ulceration*

Chlorhexidine, 0.2 to 0.5%   15 ml four times daily.
Additional advantage of inhibiting plaque formation and so preventing gingivitis where patient cannot brush teeth.

Povidone-iodine 1%   15 ml six times daily. Only for limited duration (e.g. acute viral stomatitis) due to iodine ingestion.

(e) *Astringent mouthwash for use in many forms of oral ulceration*

Zinc sulphate 1%   Diluted in four parts of water and used as required for relief of symptoms. (This preparation may have a therapeutic effect due to the action of zinc rather than to its astringency.)

(f) *Antiviral preparation, for use in shingles or herpes simplex infections spreading on to perioral skin*

Idoxuridine 5% in dimethyl sulphoxide   Painted on to vesicles four to six times daily.
(stronger solutions may be required)

(g) *Local anaesthetic preparations for discomfort arising from severe ulceration*

Lignocaine 2% solution   5 ml as a mouthrinse as required
(Xylocaine viscous and Xylotox oral solution)
Lignocaine Gel   Apply to lesions as required.

(h) *Steroid preparations for use in various disorders*

Hydrocortisone Lozenges 2.5 mg   Allowed to dissolve next to ulcerated area in aphthae and erosive lichen planus. Four lozenges per day.

Triamcinolone Dental Paste   Sparingly applied to ulcers of aphthae and erosive lichen planus four to six times daily.

Hydrocortisone solution 10%   15 ml used four times daily, for a limited duration
(usually made up from ampoules designed   only, in cases of severe aphthae, erosive lichen planus,
for injection)   erythema multiforme, pemphigus and pemphigoid.

0.5 mg Betamethasone soluble tablets		One to two tablets dissolved in 15 ml water as a mouthwash four times daily. More convenient for prescribing, and for use in same conditions as 10% hydrocortisone solution.

(i) *Sialogogue and lubricant mouthrinse used in cases of xerostomia*

Citric acid	25 g	
Glycerine	1 litre	Dilute according to taste and use as often as necessary.
Essence of lemon	40 ml	
Yellow colouring		

FURTHER READING

Cawson, R. A. & Spector, R. G. (1975) *Clinical Pharmacology in Dentistry.* Edinburgh: Churchill Livingstone.
Herxheimer, A. (1976) *Lancet,* **ii,** 1186.

INDEX

283